A MEMOIR OF DISASTER,
COMEBACKS, & FORGING A NEW PATH

YEAH, THAT WAS STUPID

JACQUES POIRIER

Published by Jacques Poirier

Printed in the United States of America

Paperback ISBN: 979-8-9898820-0-7
Hardcover ISBN: 979-8-9898820-1-4
Ebook ISBN: 979-8-9898820-2-1
Audiobook ISBN: 979-8-9898820-3-8

First Edition

CONTENTS

TO MY PARENTS, FAMILY, AND CLOSE FRIENDS, WHOSE SUPPORT WAS UNENDING IN THIS ENDEAVOR: THIS MEMOIR NEVER WOULD HAVE BEEN A REALITY WITHOUT YOUR UNWAVERING ENCOURAGEMENT.

AND TO THOSE INCREDIBLY CLOSE FRIENDS WHO WERE TAKEN TOO EARLY FROM US. YOUR MEMORY GAVE ME COURAGE TO IMPACT THE WORLD.

AUTHOR'S NOTE

While the events in this story are true, to the best of my ability to remember them, all names except my own have been changed.

PREFACE

DON'T ATTEMPT SUICIDE! Under no circumstances should you ever attempt suicide. I attempted suicide, and it ended very, very badly for me.

I wish I'd understood how bad an idea it was before making that stupid decision. I would have made a different choice if I'd known what I know today. But at the same time, I can't regret my actions. Having gone through everything I did gives me credibility when I tell people not to consider suicide as an option. Everybody who isn't suicidal says not to do it, and it may feel easy to write their opinions off because they don't know how you feel. Mine come from a place of experience.

My story is meant to provide a perspective not many people will ever get a chance to share. In my most desperate moments, compassion, wise guidance, and finally tough love enabled me to cross a bridge between despair and hope. In sharing that journey with you, my goal is to inspire those who feel the way I did to cross the bridge themselves and stand with me in this new territory.

It's a land many don't get to see. Around eight hundred thousand people die by suicide every year globally—twice the number of homicide victims. In 2017, 1.4 percent of global deaths were from suicide. In the United States, suicide rates increased by 30 percent between 2000 and 2020.[1] Even those whose lives seem perfect to others may find themselves on the wrong side of the bridge.

QUICK HEADS-UP / TRIGGER WARNING: In chapters 10, 11, and 12, I lay out everything leading up to and following my attempt. I've included all the gory details because readers need to understand the reality of what happens when somebody tries to end their own life. It's important that I stop as many people as possible from taking the path I once chose. It's truly not worth it.

ON A FINAL NOTE, we're all different individuals facing different circumstances, and *I don't have all the solutions*! You'll likely have to look a little further for help and information after reading my account, and that's okay.

SUICIDE HOTLINE

SUICIDEPREVENTIONLIFELINE.ORG

1-800-273-8255

1 Daniel C. Ehlman et al., "Changes in Suicide Rates—United States, 2019 and 2020," *Morbidity and Mortality Weekly Report* 71, no. 8 (February 2022): 306–312, http://dx.doi.org/10.15585/mmwr.mm7108a5external icon.

1 WIPEOUT

I WAS PUSHED to the crest of a large hill. My excitement grew as my father and I neared the top, cruising confidently past the oak and maple trees that decorated our neighbors' perfectly manicured lawns. It felt like nature called to me in alluring shades of greens, browns, yellows, and blacks. This would be my shining moment—the moment when I learned to ride a bicycle. I was eager to get from one side of the road to the other. Ready to look cool.

As I prepared for launch, my father looked at me solemnly and motioned for me to get off the bike. He knelt, held out a wrench, and got to work. *Wait, what are you doing,* I thought. *This wasn't part of the deal.* Before I knew it, four wheels had become two.

In hindsight, I should've seen this coming. While my mother believed that my brother and I were cut from a perfect stone, flawless from birth, my father believed that perfection had to be earned. Helping us earn it—and proving our awesomeness to the world—was his job. A big part of that involved turning me into an athletic machine as quickly as humanly possible. He had insisted that I learn how to swim (involving many trips with my mom to the YMCA) and ski (involving many trips with my mom to Perfect North Slopes) while I was still learning to talk. My first attempt at skiing had resulted in me falling headfirst in the snow. My mom had to help me stand, as I couldn't do it on my own. After a few failures, I was finally able to move downhill without tumbling, and when I did, my mother smiled at me proudly. With rosy cheeks, chapped lips, and tears running down my face due to the cold, I didn't want to show weakness. I stood up tall despite aching all over.

So it made sense that, at age three, I was going to begin my career as a professional cyclist before I knew how to take a piss in the toilet without missing the seat. Training wheels were not an option.

"Hop on," my dad said. Before I knew it, I felt a nudge from behind. Shit, I wasn't crossing from one side of the road to the other—I was going downhill. Okay, I was scared now. Not quite ready to be a man yet. *I admit defeat! Grab me!* When nobody did, I thought, *I'm going to die.*

Forgetting what brakes were, I went careening down the hill at the speed of light and crashed through several thornbushes. A few leaves ended up in my mouth, but those bushes were no match for my out-of-control momentum. I continued over a dirt ledge, collided with a wooden fencepost, landed deeper in the woods, and flipped over the handlebars *Jackass 2.0*–style. A second set of thorn bushes, much taller and thornier than the first, slowed my final descent.

Maybe twenty numb seconds after I hit the ground, the shock wore off. Tears ran down my cheeks as I began to feel the scrapes and bruises that covered my entire body and the wooden splinters that had ended up in my knee after I'd split the fencepost in half. I had been defeated by nature for the first time.

I looked behind me. A large man was sprinting down the hill in my direction. My father had never moved so quickly in his life. His tumbling mass of protein and carefully sculpted muscle followed the bicycle tracks that had sent me over the cliff—or at least what seemed like a cliff to a three-year-old. That was my cue. By the time my father made it to the bottom of the hill and witnessed the carnage, I had to convey a sense of badassery. Weakness was not in the family name.

Inside, I was a bag of tears. But I quit crying, stood up , and shook off the sweat and blood as if I performed Evel Knievel–worthy stunts every day of my life.

My father looked proud.

2 CHARISMA AND CONSEQUENCES

DON'T GET THE wrong idea. When my parents weren't encouraging me to pick fights with gravity, my early childhood was happy and fulfilling. I lived in a house with gardens in the front and back, and I loved everything in them, from the rosebushes to the lavender bushes to my favorite of all, the puffballs. The puffballs, which I referred to as exploding mushrooms, were fun to kick. It always irritated my mom when I did it right next to her as she tended the garden, and the dust coated everything close to it.

The world beyond my front yard felt just as welcoming. Indiana was a beautiful state, and I loved the scenery. I followed a comfortable routine—going to classes at a nearby private Catholic school, attending church on Wednesdays, and playing soccer on weekends. Generally speaking, I enjoyed my life, and on the rare occasion that I encountered adverse circumstances, it was usually my own fault.

Like the booger incident, for instance.

Most of my early school days were spent drawing in class and playing a game called "the monster" during recess. The worst thing that could happen was getting yelled at for not paying attention. On this particular day, however, I found myself sitting in a dark corner of my kindergarten class, facing the walls. I glanced back to see thirty pairs of eyes staring at me, my red nose, and my dunce cap. The class started yelling and laughing uncontrollably. Her voice rising over the noise, Miss Maddox instructed me not to pick my nose and wipe it on another student. If I ever did it again, she said, I'd be plopped in a different corner and fitted with another unique, well-decorated dunce cap.

The teacher's reprimand shocked me. After all, my mom never seemed to mind the boogers I'd deposited on her couch and spread along the underside of her kitchen table. Maybe she enjoyed the free decoration. Actually, now that I think about it, she never did catch me. But that didn't occur to me then. All I knew was that I had been punished for doing something that was completely acceptable at home.

Really, I wasn't used to dealing with negative consequences for any of my actions. My mom let me get away with quite a bit when I was that age, and she came to my rescue every time somebody dared try punishing me. The booger incident was no exception. After I told her everything, she waltzed right into that school and chewed Miss Maddox out for what seemed like hours. There was no escaping her wrath.

But an issue arose. While my mom may have been able to intimidate my teacher into backing off, she couldn't do the same thing with every classmate who'd witnessed my abject humiliation. I had to do something to salvage my reputation and regain their approval.

A solution came to me courtesy of the movie *A Christmas Story*, which I'd watched with my family a few weeks after Christmas. In one hilarious scene, two boys approach a group of kids and triple-dog dare one of them to lick an ice-covered pole. The kid's tongue sticks to the pole, and an ambulance has to be called to extract him.

So I thought it would be a bright idea to follow in this character's footsteps. In the days following my banishment to the corner, I attempted to impress three of the coolest girls in my class, telling them about the scene and offering to reenact it for them on the playground. They were not impressed, to say the least—and in any case, there weren't any cold poles around to help me demonstrate my comedic prowess. It was time to up the ante.

"Triple-dog dare me to do *anything* and I'll do it."

"I dare you to eat a worm," the tallest girl said.

Challenge accepted. Digging in the cold soil, I uncovered the bodies of two earthworms. I grabbed the largest one, which was half a foot long, put it in my palm, and ate it. No hesitation. The girls all cried and ran away.

My grand gesture had failed. Instead of wooing the cool girls, I'd ended up with an incurable case of cooties. Sadly, this wouldn't be the last time I'd reach for an over-the-top solution that only made the problem worse.

3 LEGOS AND LOSSES

CREATIVITY WAS ALWAYS one of my strong suits. In addition to drawing when I was supposed to be listening to the teacher, I was the world's biggest Lego fanatic. I loved wielding those multi-shaped pieces of plastic, manifesting mighty works out of nothing.

I was sitting on the Lego-covered floor in our large living room, working on one of my masterpieces, just before life as I knew it entered an alternate dimension. Nothing seemed amiss as I toiled between the two chairs draped in inexpensive brown leather and a huge, early '90s television set. The now-archaic TV probably weighed a little more than the heavyweight about to be dropped on my six-year-old mind, but only a little.

As I clicked the bricks into place, I heard a knock at the door and sat up straighter. Who would be visiting us now? It was the Sunday night after Thanksgiving, and we weren't expecting any more guests. My mother seemed less surprised. She looked through the window, and her expression told me that whoever it was, she'd been waiting for them to arrive for a while.

She opened the door, and my father stepped onto the doormat. I got excited when I realized it was him—I'd been told he was away on business—but I was quickly distracted by my Legos.

A heated discussion ensued. I had no clue as to what they were arguing about. I didn't know why my mom was crying or why my dad was yelling at her. She was always pretty noisy, so maybe he was mad at her for being noisy? Whatever the reason, it freaked me out a little to hear them go at each other like that. But I didn't do anything to call attention to the fact that I was in earshot of the whole thing. Three years after flipping over my handlebars, I'd gotten very good at hiding fear. I sat there quietly until my father left the porch of our old home while my mother tried hard to hide her tears.

The divorce proceedings started shortly after that.

• • • • • • •

The abrupt (from my perspective) dissolution of my parents' marriage was followed by the rapid expansion of my immediate family. My dad remarried within a year of the divorce. My mom remarried a year and a half after that, bringing the household where I spent most of my time from three to six people: my younger brother, Lucas, and I gained a stepdad and two stepsiblings, Emily and Matt. Emily was older than me, Matt slightly younger by a couple years. Every other weekend, Lucas and I stayed at my dad's place, where I'd hang out in my room and play on the PlayStation, not coming out for much of anything besides meals.

Throughout the upheaval and adjustment, my maternal grandfather played an important role in my life. Big family trips to Mississippi to see Grandpa were common, and I loved being around him. He was like a better-looking version of Rodney Dangerfield—very personable, always telling jokes, the life of any party. He loved music and introduced me to the Beach Boys, one of my favorite bands to this day. Despite having a headstrong nature, he was a hard person to get into an argument with. He had a knack for diffusing tense situations, and he was calm and patient regardless of what was going on around him. Seven of us grandkids could be in the room screaming our heads off and he wouldn't bat an eye—unlike my mom, who'd be freaking out over all the commotion.

When I was eleven, we stayed at my uncle's house on the bayou, not far from Grandpa. Uncle Jerry was every bit as funny as my grandfather, always telling jokes. In fact, I could never tell when he was being serious, because he always acted like he was joking. Being around him was always a good time.

During this particular visit, however, my mother and I got into a big argument the night we arrived. I wanted to play with the handheld videogame I'd brought. While I genuinely enjoyed the company of my immediate and extended family, I also liked doing my own thing without interruption. My mom wanted me to put the electronics away, be more social, and behave like a more responsible human.

I never enjoyed being told what to do. Probably no kid does. But prior to the divorce, my inclination had been to suck it up and follow whatever directives my parents handed down. After they split, I was confused as to why any of what was happening was happening, and my distress manifested as open rebellion. It pissed me off when my mom ordered me to clean this up, pick that up. When she tried to force me to complete tasks and do chores, I became combative with her.

I should mention here that the emotional state that caused me to act out didn't go unnoticed by my parents. I may have been reluctant to show weakness or fear, but I had no interest in hiding the fact that I was upset. Concerned about my well-being after they'd resettled us into our respective blended families, they decided that we—Mom and Dad, my brother, my stepsister, and my stepbrother—should all go to family counseling.

The counseling was kind of useless. The whole point was for me to get in touch with my emotions, I guess, but I didn't really understand what was going on, and I didn't know what I was doing there. The therapist would ask me how I felt about something, offering different possible answers, and I had no idea how to respond. My parents ended up trying to fill in the blanks based on whatever experiences they'd had with me. It was as if I were taking multiple-choice tests on my psyche and getting a D-minus every time. The whole thing felt like a chore. I just wanted to go home and play with my Legos.

At any rate, the three or so years of therapy didn't provide me with the kinds of emotional-regulation skills that would've come in handy the night of the big argument. It escalated to the point where a tear ran down my mother's face, which completely baffled me. Why was this strong woman crying over something so silly? We'd had dozens of fights like this, and she'd never responded that way. *I cried a million times because of her telling me what to do,* I told myself. *She doesn't deserve sympathy for her tears.*

I essentially told her to shut up. And she did. Until she muttered something I could barely make out.

"This is the last time you're probably ever going to see your grandpa, and you don't want to spend any time with us?"

Her words passed over me like a breeze. My grandpa had been a pilot during World War II and received several commendations for his bravery. He was energetic and strong and still had a full head of hair—he could never be worn down by age. Instead of acknowledging or even stopping to consider what my mother had told me, I screamed, threw a temper tantrum like an out-of-control child, and retreated to a corner of the house to be alone.

Fireworks began outside, and I could hear the pulsating and vibration of the rockets from where I sat. My mother walked into the room and encouraged me to come out and take a family photo with everyone. I refused. I was distraught and upset with her, and I felt like the best retribution was to absent myself from the photo. I said less than ten words to my grandfather the entire night.

Despite all the energy I put into my little insurrection, I didn't think about the incident much after we left Mississippi. Life went on, and I had more pressing matters to think about. For instance, the piano recital that was coming up in a few months.

Like a lot of kids, I took piano lessons because my parents made me, putting in thirty to forty-five minutes of practice every day. I didn't have any natural talent, and I never really got good at it. Every time I practiced or sat down for a lesson, I couldn't wait to be done. It was boring as hell. But I kept plugging away in preparation for the recital.

Finally, the big night arrived. The whole family came to see the results of all my dutiful if unenthusiastic work. I wasn't nervous—getting in front of people was never a problem for me—but I also wasn't particularly excited. I just wanted to get it over with so I could go home and play Halo.

My turn came, and I played a duet with my instructor. I don't remember much about the performance itself, probably because I had no emotional investment in it whatsoever. What I do remember is the trip home. I basked in the praise of my siblings, who were crammed into the back seat of our minivan with me, my mother, and my stepfather. For the first fifteen minutes, our drive was filled with laughter and joy.

Then my mother's phone rang, and the happy notes shifted into a minor key. The car became quiet as she spoke in hushed tones, clearly trying not to cry. After the three-minute call, she announced that my grandpa had died that evening in his sleep.

My grandfather's presence had provided a sense of continuity when everything else in my life felt chaotic. He'd been one of my most important role models. Now he was gone, and I could only process one thought: How could I have been so selfish as to not take a picture with *him* when I was only upset with my mother? That question cycled through my mind over and over again for the rest of the year.

My grandfather's death was the first to teach me that someone you love, cherish, and respect might not be in your life tomorrow. I'd thought he was invincible, but he wasn't. No one is.

4 CRACKED SHELLS AND CONSEQUENCES

HIGH SCHOOL WAS pretty uneventful. While I wasn't reserved or antisocial by any stretch of the imagination, I focused most of my attention on cross-country sports and schoolwork. Credit for my diligence went mostly to my mother, who wanted me to study all the time. Having gotten over my rebellious phase, I'd come to terms with her high standards and followed the rules that she laid out.

I graduated with decent grades and made it into Indiana University / Bloomington as a member of the Army ROTC program. While I was aware that IU was a top-10 party school, I was expecting the same daily grind I'd experienced in high school. My college career would consist of school, sports, homework, and then sleep, over and over again until graduation.

I'd never been so wrong about anything in my life.

After my parents helped me with the move-in process, I walked through the halls, getting to know the other guys on my floor.

Everybody was out and about, knocking on doors and socializing. I ended up hanging out and talking with a small group of people for a couple of hours. One of them told us that his sister was friends with the girlfriend of one of the frat brothers at a fraternity whose name I'll omit to protect the innocent (and guilty). If we pretended to know the frat brother, he said, we could get into the big party they were throwing.

We got through the door no problem, then went our separate ways to experience our first taste of college life. I started ripping shots and ended up conversing with a woman who was twenty-two. I never did get her name. Or at least I don't remember getting it. I'd never partied in high school and was a total lightweight at this point, so the evening was kind of a blur.

Talk turned to more than talk, and we ended up in somebody's bedroom. I started asking her a question after our brief sexual encounter had more or less concluded, but she interrupted me. She had a boyfriend, she explained, and I needed to go. Right that second. The boyfriend had just walked up the stairs and was heading in the direction of our room.

I ravaged several shots of alcohol while sprinting toward a door, then jumped into the closet and hid. Too bad it wasn't a bathroom, as I really needed one. Eventually I just peed in the closet. After fifteen minutes, when the coast was finally clear, I left.

I met two foreign exchange students while walking back to my dorm. As I was still relatively thirsty, they mentioned that they had a bottle of vodka, and I joined them. I kid you not, twenty people were shoved together like sardines in their tiny dorm room. I took several more shots and continued to make new friends. By the end of the night, I'd drunk more than I had during four years of high school.

The entire experience was a revelation. I'd thought my routine at home, utterly devoid of adventure, had been typical. Was I unusually sheltered because my mom never let me do anything crazy? Or was going off the rails like this new to every college freshman? Either way, I felt exhilarated. My four years of being complacent, of being confined within a safe little eggshell, were over. The risks I'd faced during my first night on my own had rewarded me with a deluge of endorphins, and it was what I'd been waiting for my entire life.

• • • • • • •

For those of you who aren't familiar with ROTC, the Reserve Officers' Training Corps, it's a training program where you volunteer your time to become a cadet during your four years as an undergraduate. After graduation, instead of trying to find a job, you either enlist in the reserves or go active duty. Your branch is selected for you based on grades, performance within the program, fitness, and how well you do at a summer training course between your junior and senior years. A lot is expected of cadets, and I knew I would have to focus on my grades and excel at my studies if I was to succeed.

As days turned into weeks, I developed new friendships through ROTC and, as it happened, several were members of Chi Gamma Zeta Beta, one of the fraternities on campus. Two of them, Bob and Bill, were looking for people with similar goals and attitudes to join, and they invited me to a little get-together at the house one weekend early in the semester. Over the course of the next couple of months, they continued to recruit me, and I eventually decided that pledging was in my best interest. The group of thirty guys in the house right outside fraternity row were like a mini-community. I had never participated in anything quite like it. Membership gave me an opportunity to become a leader on campus, and it felt incredible to be a part of something larger than myself.

Contrary to popular belief, there was no hazing during the eight-week pledging period. Why not? It could have been due to the nature of the men involved. When your fraternity mainly has army cadets in it, there's a significant emphasis on integrity and not violating people's boundaries. I was never asked to do anything I felt uncomfortable doing. I engaged in some heavy-duty partying for sure, but all of it was on my own initiative. After so many years of studying hard and following my mother's rules, prevented from doing all the exciting things I'd come to assume everyone else got to do when they were fifteen or sixteen, I needed to make up for lost time. It was imperative that I live my college life on my own terms.

I enjoyed every moment I got to spend with my brothers in the fraternity. Still, it seemed like some key component was missing. Getting all of my entertainment and gratification from large events and parties left little time for pursuing loftier goals, or even figuring out what those goals might be. It felt empty. I kept losing ground in the academic realm while everyone else around me moved forward. It was so hard to keep up when distractions lurked around every corner. I thought I had the ability to make good choices, given that I'd developed decent study habits in high school, but I allowed chaos to consume my daily routine. The only thing that had changed was that I had the freedom to do whatever I wanted. This was unfamiliar territory.

Things came to a head on Halloween, the biggest night of the year for us. We planned on having several hundred people over that night—the night before I needed to take tests in three different classes. I was definitely not ready for them. But my Scuba Steve costume with a custom mini-keg on my back in lieu of an oxygen tank took priority. I drank myself into a deep stupor. As I was dropped off in front of my freshman dorm, whoever drove me there asked, "Hey, you gonna make it up there all right?"

"Yeah, yeah, yeah, get the fuck out of here," I said with great confidence.

I barely made it up three flights of stairs. By the time I got to the second story, I was crawling. Crawling turned to slithering, and eventually I entered, slow and steady. When I finally made it to the third floor, I rushed to the bathroom, took off the wetsuit that was part of my costume, and expelled an avalanche of vomit all over a sink and urinal.

Stephanie, our hall's resident assistant, walked by the bathroom at some point after I'd emptied the contents of my stomach, walked past me, then did a double take and stepped back.

"You okay in there?"

"Yeah," I muttered, "I, uh, I'm tooty groody."

When Stephanie was a safe distance away, I rushed back to my room before she could witness the entrails of puke along the floor. I turned my doorknob and flung the door open. Home base at last. I'd passed through the eternal gate and made it through to the other side. Relief beset me until I heard several knocks.

Apparently, the sounds of my groaning could be heard echoing through the hall, and Stephanie had returned to check on my well-being. Everything went quite black after she entered the room. Ten minutes later, she woke me up. A university cop stood next to her, holding out an underage drinking citation for me to sign.

Well, that sucks was the first thing that popped into my mind. Not *Man, I hope I'll be okay in the morning,* or *Good thing they're not escorting me to the police station.* I passed out with the ticket in my hand.

Seeing fourteen missed calls on my phone the next morning was more than enough to sober me up. My mother and father had been informed of the incident, and they were furious.

But oh, it got better. At the end of the semester, soon after I finished my drinking citation classes, my grades were released. I got two calls on the same day—one from my lieutenant colonel and one from my parents. I was millimeters away from losing my scholarship. My citation alone had the potential to destroy my standing in the ROTC program, and my GPA, 2.6, was low enough for them to put me on academic probation. To make things even worse, I might not be able to become a full-fledged member of the fraternity I'd been pledging to for months.

Freedom had proven to be too much for me to handle. Now I had no choice but to plug in and atone for all the previous semester's damage. No more parties, no more drinking during the week, and no putting off studying for the test until the night before. I lost half of the "friends" I'd gained during semester one. XYZ allowed me to join on the condition that my next set of grades be above a 3.0 average. I got a 3.1. It was too close for comfort.

Sadly, I learned nothing from that experience. After my semester of drudgery, I devised a plan that I believed would enable me to party while maintaining decent grades and completing my Army ROTC requirements: I would work hard on my school obligations one week and do the opposite the next. By my primitive calculations, the former would neutralize the latter.

I put my plan into action at the beginning of my sophomore year. Juggling chaos became my new hobby.

5 THE CALL TO (STUPID) ADVENTURE

I STARED AT the computer screen in the library, reading an article about the West Indies for a summer class, Jamaican and Caribbean Culture 301. For once, I wasn't distracted by thoughts of the next party, the clicking of fingers on keyboards from the dozen or so other students sitting at their computers, or anything else. Fully absorbed, I took in the information regarding wealth disparities among various Caribbean countries.

I was twenty at this point, a second-semester sophomore, and this was first time I'd connected emotionally with anything related to coursework in a while. Something about the descriptions of how people in the West Indies lived spoke to me. I wanted to involve myself in this area of the world. While I had no clue how I might accomplish that, a seed had been planted.

Some weeks later, I sat in front of a different computer screen, indulging in my chewing-tobacco addiction. Staring at the can of chew prompted a stream of seemingly inconsequential thoughts.

Black chewing tobacco.

Can.

Can is empty now.

No more tobacco.

Empty tin can.

Where can I get more?

What if I can't get more?

Wait, what if there was none left?

What if everyone had empty tin cans that had no food?

What place exists in the Caribbean where no food is left?

Can I go there?

And boom! A switch flipped in my head and it all came together. I was going to plan a trip to one of the largest slum cities in the world, Cite Soleil.

Three years earlier, in 2010, an earthquake had struck Haiti, killing 250,000 people in the blink of an eye. Homes were devastated, lives irrevocably changed. The country's GDP was already low on a global scale, but it had been about average for that part of the world. After the earthquake, this beautiful but barely stable nation-state became one of the poorest in the Caribbean, and they still hadn't recovered. But I could help them . . . somehow. I'd wanted to do something exceptional from the time I was very young, had always wanted to be of service to others in need, but didn't know how. Cite Soleil, Haiti, was my opportunity, my calling.

When I think back on it, there was no logical reason for me to fixate on this location. If I wanted to help people in poverty, there was no shortage of places to do it. I wouldn't even have to leave my home state. But convenience wasn't the point, and neither was logic. I wanted an adventure.

For months, the bizarro version of a work-life balance I'd crafted—studying hard one week and partying hard the next—had provided me with a steady supply of excitement. Could I finish all of my assignments while hungover? Would I be able to pass my classes after putting off work until the last possible minute? Pushing the limits of my abilities made every exam, every deadline, feel like a cliffhanger. The problem was that after over a semester of living this way, it had become routine. Unfulfilling. Now I yearned for something new to keep me on the edge of my seat, a different way to harness my impulsivity and desire for change.

Haiti had everything I thought I needed. Turmoil. Constant action. A large number of underprivileged people who were just waiting for someone like me to offer assistance. And I felt a profound connection to them. The earthquake that had transformed their lives, bringing their standard of living from average to nothing, called to mind the turbulence of my own emotional and scholastic descent. It was ridiculous of me to compare the consequences of my self-imposed lifestyle with the suffering of these people—I realize this now—but at the time it felt justified. My routine needed to be disrupted. Traveling to an infinitely more interesting location and placing myself in a precarious situation would provide the surge of adrenaline I needed, the antidote to the monotony of my life.

I went down the rabbit hole watching documentaries on how people had lived on less than a dollar a day in this country. I wanted to duplicate the experience, immersing myself in the lives of the citizens who'd been affected by natural disaster. By the end of April, my research was finished and it was time to act. I ordered the plane tickets, packed a rucksack, and prepped for a solid week. All systems were go; I was ready for anything that might happen. Being a self-reliant person, I found it easy to do all of this on my own. The hard part was keeping it a secret. As far as my family knew, I was coming home for the summer.

So a few days after school concluded in May, I was sitting in the Indianapolis International Airport. In ten minutes I would board a plane to Chicago, then another plane to Fort Lauderdale, and then take two other connecting flights to Haiti. The moment of truth had arrived: it was time to let my family in on the plan.

I called my mom first. To my surprise, Mark, my stepdad, answered her phone. I told him what I was doing. He took it about as well as you'd expect. After telling me to stop and think about my actions, and to not get on the plane, he handed the phone to my mother.

I restated my plan. Dead silence ensued while she processed a ridiculous number of emotions and thought about whether she was going to cry, scream, or pull out her hair.

"You're joking, right?" she said after what felt like three hours.

No, I insisted. I was ready to hop on that flight and go on the biggest adventure of my life.

"Don't move; stay right there!"

I hung up, knowing exactly who she was going to dial next, and got on the plane.

Sure enough, when I landed in Chicago, I had voicemail from my father. This conversation would be easier, I thought. He loved traveling, and if anyone would appreciate the idea of a trip to an unfamiliar locale, it would be him.

Yeah, no. He was just as alarmed as my mom and stepdad, demanding that I drop the whole idea and come back to Indiana. When he failed to convince me, a buffet line of calls from my mom ensued.

"Get your fucking ass home, or we're cutting you off," she said. (My mom only cusses once in a blue moon). "Why are you running away from home? What do you plan to get out of this? Why are you doing this? What is the goal?"

"Mom, stop. Relax. I thought this through."

"Like hell you have! Go home right now."

"I can't, and I love you," I said, once again hanging up.

The calls went on and on. It was like listening to one of those revved-up clockwork toys on repeat. Finally I turned off my phone again and boarded the next plane.

When I landed at Fort Lauderdale International Airport hours later, a feeling of remorse hit me hard, multiple thoughts racing through my mind. Was my family never going to look at me the same again? I needed to think this through.

On the one hand, I found my parents' concern irrational. They couldn't see how well I'd thought everything out. I wasn't worried about my mom's talk of cutting me off, either. That was obviously an empty threat, a desperate attempt to force me to turn around and come back. It felt manipulative. But I also recognized that it came from a good place. She cared about me, she wasn't comfortable with me going to a dangerous foreign country alone, and she would do whatever it took to keep me safe. Further, she truly had no idea why I was doing this. She was missing all of the puzzle pieces that I'd spent so much time putting together beforehand, so there was no way for her to understand the full picture. The problem was that, in trying to explain it to her, my motives sounded muddied and confusing even to myself. It's difficult to explain why you're going to such great lengths to do something so risky when the real reason is that you're bored.

At this point, even though my parents had used every scare tactic they could to retrieve me, my biggest concern wasn't my own safety but their emotional well-being. Now I had to make the most important choice I'd ever made in my life: talk to my parents again before getting on the next flight, or continue, leave my phone off for the duration of my two-month trip, and take a chance on damaging my relationship with them permanently.

After hours of battling it out in my mind, I gave up and decided to turn my phone back on. There were tons of missed calls. At least twenty family members and friends had reached out. Every single person was concerned.

My mom called again as I digested the missed voicemails and text messages. She told me to come home, or I would be disowned. Felt like more of a threat at this point than a desperate plea, but I still understood her intent.

So now I faced an even heavier decision. My first option was to follow through, make the trip, and deal with the fallout when I got home, if there was a home to go back to. The second was to call the whole thing off—fifteen minutes before boarding the final plane—and regret not going for the rest of my life. *Is this who I am? The kind of person who gives up on his goals?*

I decided not to go. I was a pussy now and forever. Dammit. Time to go home.

My mom paid for my return flight, and she and my stepfather picked me up at the airport the next day. I stared at her, mad as hell, and pretty much didn't talk to her for months.

I'd made the right choice in the end. Still, I was no closer to understanding my own motives for doing the things I did, much less the effects of my behavior on others.

6 JOURNEY TO JAMAICA

MY NEXT OPPORTUNITY for a trip abroad came in the form of an academic requirement. I needed to travel to a foreign country to complete my degree in international studies, and as my junior year came to an end in 2014, five classmates and I prepared for a two-week stay in Jamaica.

The official objective of the trip, being a school trip, was educational. For three weeks prior to leaving, we would learn about our destination and pick a subject we wanted to focus on while we were there. Possible topics ranged from farming to road construction and maintenance to watershed initiatives. By August 3, we'd write a formal paper and give a presentation on the problems we identified, offering solutions based on our observations, the opinions we solicited from the people who lived there, and statistical analyses.

When our initial classwork began, I sat around a large table with the other students as we talked about why we were fascinated with Jamaica and what we hoped to gain from going. Their personalities were remarkably different from mine. While I was energetic and chatty, everyone else had a laid-back vibe. One classmate, the only guy besides me, was a clumsy, shy redhead. Another wore a dozen bracelets, each with a peace symbol on it. As the resident meathead, I stuck out like a sore thumb. During the first of four classes, I asked, "Are there going to be any gyms where we're going?" I received the ugliest stares from the women.

Three weeks later, all six of us boarded a plane with our professor, taking a direct flight to Jamaica. Eric the redhead and I sat next to each other while Professor Clarke and three of the female students sat in a single row together. Eric could not stop talking about video games, which irked the shit out of me; I had no clue as to what this guy was talking about. Not that I was judgmental or anything.

After a refreshing nap that lasted most of the five-hour flight, we touched down. From my window I stared at the most beautiful place I'd ever encountered in my life. The green landscape spread out before us like a vast ocean till the earth met the sky. Though I had never thought of myself as poetic or artistic, this place drew out all my hidden creativity. My fingers itched for a canvas and some paints, for I knew my camera could never do the scenery justice.

We were picked up by a shuttle driver and drove for another four or five hours to the country's interior toward our destination, Ambassabeth. This small village in the mountains boasted several hundred people, a bunch of horses and goats, and a river that ran through its center. It looked nothing like the touristy parts of the country shown in magazine articles and advertisements—no beaches or high-end resorts for us. I didn't care. I was awestruck by Ambassabeth's natural beauty.

If the landscape blew my mind, the people defied all of my expectations. Back when I was planning the Haiti trip, I thought I would swoop in, help people who were impoverished, and increase their happiness. They couldn't already be happy—they were destitute, right? Well, if I had to guess, the villagers in Ambassabeth, Jamaica, weren't much better off than the Haitians I'd wanted to rescue. Each child seemed to have only one toy and ten different ways of playing with it. But I quickly realized that even though they were living at subsistence level, surviving day by day on what they could produce and grow, they were happier than any other group of people I'd ever met.

Two specific individuals exemplified this state of mind. The first was a middle-aged man, Smokey, who served as a tour guide of sorts for us. Even though I couldn't understand a damn word he said in his Jamaican patois, I got along with Smokey from the moment he introduced himself to me. His handshake was confident and strong and made me feel like I'd been clamped with an industrial wrench. He had at least as many scars as I did, most of which were the result of boar bites. He could name every strand of hemp that existed. Most importantly, he had a positive attitude that the people around him responded to. He treated everyone with respect and kindness whether he knew them or not, and they reciprocated.

Smokey was our captain for the duration of our adventures, his "ship" an ancient sedan with all four doors missing, no cushions, and a tailgate that creaked and howled like a wolverine.

He's probably still driving that beauty today. On the third day of our trip, we got into that car and took a trip to the local market, a six-hundred-square-foot grocery store. There wasn't room for much else on the side of a mountain face with steep cliffs and drop-offs in the middle of the jungle. He waved at every passerby that waltzed past the car as we headed back down the mountain. Everyone smiled back, for an aura of kindness surrounded the man. As days passed, I grew to admire the way he balanced a laidback nature with a sense of responsibility. I wanted to be more like him.

The other person who made a huge impression on me was an eight-year-old named Jay. A whole flock of crazy cool kids gathered around me every chance they got—apparently they found me entertaining—but Jay looked up to me as an older brother of sorts. He followed me everywhere I went and copied whatever I did. If I tried skipping a rock across a stream, he did the same. If I roundhouse kicked a banana tree, he followed suit. And like Smokey, he was filled with pure, untamed happiness. This kid sprinted straight down a hill on day two, tripped, and rolled through the bushes like I had on my bike at three years old. But damn, he got up quicker than I had, and instead of looking like he was trying not to cry, he laughed hysterically, oblivious to the cuts on his arms and face. His mom scolded him, and he ran from her. "Jay, stop, get back here!" she yelled. He completely ignored her. Watching him go was like staring at a mirror image of myself.

As I was slowly introduced to everyone else in the town, Jay and I became best friends. Through a series of several pranks, we were able to create an astounding level of mayhem. He showed me a flower that would cause brief but uncomfortable itching if you consumed small amounts of it or placed on it your skin. The little brat tried to get me to eat it. I was a pro at this kind of stuff, however, so I didn't fall for it. I pretended to chow down to gauge his reaction, and he giggled the moment he thought I'd consumed it. That's when I knew he was full of shit.

One of the girls fell for it, though. I told him to tell my classmate Sarah that the flower would have anti-aging properties if she rubbed it on her elbow. Jay had a blast, and she had a good laugh with us after when she caught us trying to do it to another girl in our group.

The other prank took a little more preparation. We'd found a giant crab with claws the size of baseballs. Jay, Smokey, and I took a bottle of rum I'd bought at the local market out of my backpack and replaced it with the crab. When we got back shortly after dark, the backpack swung over my shoulder, the stage was set. I walked up to the door of the main cabin where my classmates were huddled and placed my backpack on the warm wooden floor. Chelsea opened the bag in anticipation of cold rum on a hot, sweaty, humid day and screeched louder than an airhorn on a train.

I don't want these stories to give you the wrong impression. Jamaica isn't some kind of utopia where the people are saints and no one experiences hardship. One of the first things I noticed on the drive to Ambassabeth was that there were tons of unfinished construction projects by the side of the road—partially built houses, office buildings, and other infrastructure. When I asked the villagers about it, they told me that different parts of the government funneled money into these projects, and whatever they saved by not completing them went back into somebody's pocket. There was also a real lack of opportunity when it came to education. Most book learning took place in little schoolhouses reminiscent of what we had in the nineteenth-century United States, and most kids had little chance of attending college once they graduated high school.

At the same time, I couldn't help but be impressed—even inspired—by the way everyone navigated these challenges. The topic I'd chosen to explore before coming to Jamaica was education. As part of my research, I spent a couple of days in the schoolhouse in Ambassabeth. The walls needed to be painted, the roof needed to be replaced, and they had little in the way of study materials. Despite their lack of resources, or maybe because of it, ordinary school supplies were more valuable than machinery in these children's eyes. Every article, every newspaper, every book was utilized more effectively than the ten books I bought in a single semester for college. It was a humbling experience. I was envious, not of the children themselves, but of their work ethic. These kids were six to twelve years old and displayed more educational ambition and drive in one week than I had in my first three college years combined.

Not that I immediately followed their example. While our stay in Jamaica was supposed to be educational, it was really one-third school trip, two-thirds vacation. When we weren't doing our field research, we literally had no responsibilities at all. I, of course, took full advantage of this fact, goofing off with Jay and spending most of my time in the woods and by the creeks. And when Smokey told me about a local boar hunt that another townsman was about to journey on, I knew I had to partake.

Boar hunting was a really big deal in the interior of Jamaica. Typically, from what I was told, a hunt could take anywhere from a day to an entire week. When I responded to Smokey's information with a level of enthusiasm that could've been measured by a seismograph, he told me I should join the group the next morning before they left. "Go talk to Jordan," he remarked. My professor didn't mind as long as we came back within a day or two.

Jordan, the tracker of the group, approached me near a hammock where my classmates and I stayed. "Go pack a bag with a couple of sandwiches," he commanded. "Steal a couple of bananas from the tree out back. Get some jeans you don't mind scuffing up and be ready to go at six o'clock tomorrow morning."

I awoke at 5:30 a.m., threw on my jeans, tank top, and backpack, and joined the party. In addition to traditional hunting spears, we brought eight dogs with us. For these villagers, dogs weren't pets but hunting animals. As bad as it sounds, they were intentionally starved from time to time so that they could become more proficient at tracking. Feeding them only once per day or every other day motivated them to catch wild animals as they were driven by instinct to nourish themselves.

What was supposed to be a quick and easy two-day jaunt turned into fifteen hours of hell. We trekked over mountains and across creeks, through needle-covered trees and soggy marshes, and by the time it was all over, we hadn't caught a single boar. All I managed to subdue were some wild bananas and Ethiopian apples. I arrived back in town sweating, drenched from head to toe, and slightly delusional and dehydrated. I thought my cardio was maxed out, and here was this local jumping ten feet across riverbeds while carrying a dog. If only I'd prepped more for the army's mile run and PT test.

As I staggered back to our home base, Jay ran up to me with arms wide open for a hug. "Ya good, ya?" Smokey yelled.

"No, I'm dying," I answered. "What the fuck. How do you guys do this?" Smokey and Jordan got a good laugh out of my anguish.

Leaving Ambassabeth and heading home wasn't easy. The town had brought me a sense of peace and tranquility. I'd forged amazing friendships with the villagers. While I'd looked forward to the trip before I got here, I'd never imagined that I wouldn't want to leave.

The plane ride back was two connected flights. After a few hours, I touched down in Indianapolis, where my mom was waiting to pick me up. I had so many stories to share with her on the car ride home, I couldn't shut up for two minutes. Had I really needed a trip to Haiti to achieve the endorphin high I was looking for? Maybe this would do.

7 ARMY, ROTC, LDAC

AS EPIC AS Jamaica had been, it wasn't the most important trip I'd take all summer. When I got back to Indiana, I had a little over a week to pack for the Leadership Development and Assessment Course. At LDAC I would spend a month in Fort Knox, Kentucky, competing with thousands of other cadets in physical fitness, strategic assessment and capability, and additional challenges that brought us to the edge of mental and physical exhaustion. The scores I received would count for 30 percent of my overall evaluation at the end of my senior year, and they would help determine what branch of the army I went into upon graduation.

To prepare, I called my cousin Lawrence, who'd been a ROTC cadet at Indiana University many years ago and received an active-duty placement in the infantry as a result of his LDAC performance. His tips and pointers put me in a good state of mind to handle any situation thrown my way. It was going to be a pain in the ass, based on what he told me, but not necessarily difficult. I couldn't wait to show that I was capable of living up to the standards he'd set—maybe even exceeding them.

Another cadet from Indiana University and I carpooled to Fort Knox, chewing tobacco and mentally prepping ourselves for what was to come. We arrived at the camp several hours later, and somebody immediately started barking orders at us. I didn't let the pressure extinguish my excitement. I was confident after the call with my cousin, and I felt like I was able to take on the world.

"Fall in line, grab your gear, and check it off the list, hurry! Go! Go! Go!" Sergeant Rottweiler commanded.

"Yes, sergeant!" I responded. "Wait, which line am I getting into?"

"Jesus Christ!" he yelled, even louder than before. "Cadet, follow the tape!"

"Yes, sergeant! Wait, which colored tape?" I mumbled.

"I'm going to lose my shit, cadet. The fucking yellow ones!"

"Okay."

"Okay? It's 'Yes, sergeant!"

"Oh shit. I meant yes, sergeant! I apologize, sergeant!" I said hesitantly, more nervous now. Our on-campus training had been much tamer than this.

"Grab your gear once it's all accounted for and step into formation!" Sergeant Rottweiler ordered. My legs swooshed into place faster than my mind could process. I dropped my bag at my feet, and we proceeded to the barracks and got situated in our bunks.

The following two weeks primarily involved field training. We began with strategy and simulations. At 3:00 one morning, we took turns staying awake and watching perimeters, prepping for any fake Op 4 insurgents that could breach our theoretical position at any moment.

"Good job, Cadet Poirier! Way to get into position and respond appropriately!" Sergeant Jenkins shouted. "But next time, make sure you watch the right. You're fucking dead. That insurgent twenty feet from you has you in his sights. Switch, next person on fireguard duty, watch the perimeter, don't get your battle buddies killed."

Although the various sergeants yelled at me for an entire week about everything I screwed up, they all applauded me at the end of field training and strategy. Rifle work was next.

"You have a single target in front!" Sergeant Jenkins proclaimed. "The first clip from your M16 will be semiauto. Switch to single on the second clip. We will take turns and repeat!"

My accuracy was comparable to that of a professional dart thrower, my grouping perfect with every shot. Accolades were thrown at me left and right from every sergeant on our firing line. As you might imagine, my confidence was skyrocketing. I was destroying training.

"You're closer to being a great leader, Cadet Poirier," Sergeant Jenkins said softly. "Just don't let it go to your head."

The physical fitness test was next on the agenda at week three. I had been prepping for it throughout college. This would be my shining moment.

"Proceed to the starting line and prepare for the mile run. Stretch, do what you must do to get ready, cadets!" Sergeant Allen yelled. This was it.

I stepped up to the line and focused on the horizon. My shoes shifted as I took one step closer to the white marker. The popgun fired, signaling that it was time for me to sprint out of the gate like a racehorse.

I was panting at three quarters of a mile, but I got through the finish line in under six minutes. Yes! I killed it! The only thing left was the easy push-up and sit-up portion of the test, and I nailed those with ease as well. While other cadets were crying after not placing where they wanted to in the mile run or outright failing portions of the test, I was trying not to look as cocky as I felt. I could do anything now. All that remained was the strategy portion.

The previous three weeks had tested the limits of our physical capabilities. This last week—the most crucial part of training—would challenge our mental endurance. We needed to prove that we could make sound decisions and formulate battle plans for engagements with enemy forces in a variety of situations. We would learn four different modes of engagement: ambush, move to encounter, engagement, and recon to engagement. The last one, recon to engagement, was the hardest to pull off. How would we do if we had to approach and engage the enemy head-on? What would be the easiest way to set up an ambush for insurgents? How would we split up the squads, and where would they be placed? Would recon units be part of our preparation?

At the end of the week, we were each tested on a specific engagement model. We had to quickly draw up a battle map on the dirt floor beneath a large tent using sticks, stones, and plastic bottles—objects that would realistically be available to us on an actual battlefield. In five minutes, the cadet would draw the map. In another five minutes, they would devise a plan. And in the next five minutes, they would simulate the engagement. These last five minutes were the most important part of the entire training camp. I couldn't wait to demonstrate my critical thinking skills and thrust them into action.

I was third in line. The two cadets ahead of me left the tent one after another looking scared and confused. Was this really going to be as easy as I thought? *Yes, it is,* I told myself. *Don't overthink it, and don't let the other guys' reactions mess with your head. Get in there and prove that your success in the first three weeks can be replicated here.*

"Good luck, bro," The second cadet said to me as I approached the tent. That had to be the least confident *good luck, bro* I'd ever received.

I opened the flap and faced two sergeants I didn't recognize. Both had stern expressions on their faces.

"Get into position, cadet. This is serious. Do what you need to do. You're planning a recon to engagement," Sergeant Serious Face informed me confidently. I gulped. Fuck, seriously, the hardest engagement type? The only one I'd hoped they wouldn't test me on?

"We chose this one because we believed you could handle it," the other sergeant said. "You have five minutes to prep, go."

The first five minutes passed with significant success. My recon deployment was in place on a fake ridge. Both of my squads were in place on the flanks, ready to respond to unforeseen circumstance from every angle. I remembered the 3:00 a.m. situation from earlier in the training and replicated the tactic of switching members of each squad so that we could effectively engage if a dangerous circumstance arose. Five more minutes down, and I was ready to start the engagement. No follies yet! But these last five minutes were the most critical part of the entire plan. I couldn't mess it up now; fake green army men's lives were in my hands.

Five minutes later, I exited the tent and let out a huge sigh of relief. "Congratulations, Cadet Poirier, you kept everyone alive and had a major success with the engagement. You can go sit with the other cadets now."

I'd nailed it! No way my cadre and instructors back home would have anything bad to say about my performance!

On the last day we packed our gear, did another check, and prepped to leave the camp. All of us were congratulated for passing the training. The cadet I'd carpooled with approached me and asked how I did.

"Dude, I mastered it all. I'm excited," I proclaimed. "How did you do?"

"Eh, we'll see."

When we returned to our campus ROTC office at the end of the summer, I was told that I'd completed the camp with an E rating—I was in the top 10 percent of cadets in terms of evaluation and critiques. Success! All my prep for the camp had been worth it.

• • • • • • •

My senior year of college arrived, and with it the moment of truth. Now we would find out who received active-duty assignments and who ended up in the reserves. Most cadets in our department wanted active duty. The pay was a lot better than we'd get as paper-and-pen pushers in the States, and the excitement would be next-level.

In November, we sat at assigned tables at the ROTC Gala to receive our assignments for reserve, active-duty, and sub-branch placements within one of sixteen different branches of the army. The preferred branches were infantry and armor. In infantry (my first choice), you'd lead a platoon of ground forces, anywhere from thirty to forty-five soldiers, in an active combat zone. Armor (my second choice) involved driving and operating battle tanks like an M-1 Abrams and light infantry support vehicles.

"Cadet, please come to the front."

I took my place in line. Excitement overwhelmed me. My performance at LDAC would easily give me the edge I needed to get the placement I desired.

"Cadet Poirier, please come up."

I took the envelope containing the next four years of my life and opened it.

"Congratulations, Cadet Poirier."

My world crumbled around me.

I'd gotten reserves instead of active duty. To add insult to injury, they'd placed me in the chemical branch— no offense to anyone in that branch, I just had zero interest in it. The entire reason I'd joined ROTC was to encase myself in action abroad after college. The chemical branch would require me to play with carbon dioxide at a desk and clean N95 masks for those who'd be doing the real action. *Seriously? This boring fucking shit?* I took several deep breaths and thought, *Please tell me this is a joke!*

The paper with my reserves assignment slipped through my fingers and fell to the floor. The only thing I could do was pick it up, smile, and pretend I was happy. "Next, cadet, come on up!"

Everyone around me was smiling. Almost everyone had gotten active duty except for me. *What just happened?*

But I knew the answer. I'd come up with a strategy that I thought would compensate for all the partying that consumed me in my first year of university life. I believed my 3.1 GPA, in tandem with my fantastic LDAC score and excellent physical fitness scores, would be high enough. But several semesters of clowning around had destroyed my chances of getting the placement I wanted. It was my fault. I did this to myself.

I was one of the last cadets to leave the Gala room. As several others finished their drinks and walked out the double doors to the main hall, I remained alone. One Cadre member—an instructor in the ROTC program—came over to my table to talk to me. He'd seen this kind of thing play out before and immediately knew what was wrong. My eyes, face, and mind went blank as he asked me if I was okay. Of course, he knew I wasn't. But there was nothing he could do about it.

"Cadet. I know what you're thinking right now," Captain Summers said.

"Is this a prank?" I asked. "What do I do now?"

"No. I just want you to know that your position matters as well. You will be serving the country and saving lives in your own way," he said, tiptoeing across the edge of bullshit.

"Yeah." That was all I could say.

8 PLAN OF DISTRACTION

I DIDN'T COMPLETELY fall apart. Not right away, at least. In the weeks following the Gala, Beverly Miller kept me from succumbing to total despair. I had been dating Bev for several months, and she had a way of convincing me that anything could be overcome. She wasn't upset with my reserves placement. In fact, she was happy for me.

"I want you to quit talking about what you think of as a failure in ROTC," she told me a week after I received my placement. She gave me a cute smile. "You're not a failure. You're capable of so much outside of that stupid program."

"I know. Can we talk about something else then?" I said.

"That's what I wanted to bring up." Her smile shone even brighter. "I love you, and I love where this is going. When we move in together next year, where do you want to go?"

I laughed. "I didn't know we were moving in together."

"Yeah, well, I think it would be good for both of us," she said. "Let me look at locations, and we'll put a plan together. Just give me a couple of months to organize it."

So it wasn't like my life was terrible, or that I had nothing to look forward to after graduation, or even that anybody gave me a hard time about what had gone down. My mother and stepfather knew about the Gala results, and the only thing my mother said to me about it was that she was proud of me, and that we needed to figure out what I'd be doing next year other than the military, since reservists only serve one weekend a month, two weeks per year. Still, I felt ashamed and humiliated and didn't want her to tell anyone else that I hadn't made active duty. Her side of the family was full of veterans going back to the Revolutionary War, including my grandmother. Lawrence, my cousin who'd given me the LDAC pointers, couldn't find out that I'd failed either. Knowing I wouldn't follow in his footsteps gave me an awful feeling in my gut.

I had let them all down!

• • • • • • •

Although I mourned the loss of my dreams, I didn't want to spend the rest of my senior year moping. *One failure will not stop me from excelling in every other category of life*, I decided. Positive thinking was key. If I maxed out every other endeavor I pursued, it would distract me from my ROTC defeat, maybe even make up for it. I needed to fill what little time I had left at IU with accomplishments, leave at least a little legacy before I graduated. *I will say yes to every opportunity*, I resolved.

And I did. In my quest to distract myself, focusing my attention on anything that had nothing to do with my placement, I landed on two all-encompassing areas of interest: the Little 500 and weightlifting.

The Little 500 is the largest collegiate bicycle race in the country. Modeled after the Indy 500, it takes place at Indiana University Bloomington every May, and the money raised goes toward a scholarship fund for IU students. The cyclists in the men's race do two hundred relay-style laps around a racetrack, competing for first, second, and third place.

Even qualifying to participate is incredibly challenging. Forty- to fifty-four-member teams compete for one of the thirty-three slots for the race. A quarter of them don't make it. I had been on the Little 500 team for my fraternity during both my freshman and sophomore years. It was a big commitment, requiring us to stay away from alcohol most weekends. Our team wasn't the best by any means, but we worked our asses off.

Practice was every single day. The five of us took it seriously, as we were underdogs. We trained most mornings at 6:00 a.m. and every evening at 6:00 or 7:00 p.m. Each session lasted an hour to an hour and a half. It was grueling and required a lot of stamina built up from individual training during the winter. We were prepared, though, and made the most of each session. After four weeks, we cut our team to four for the race, leaving the fifth to work the pits. I made the team.

You'd think that this exhausting routine, on top of my classwork and ROTC obligations, would be enough to keep me occupied. In fact, it only was the tip of the iceberg. My other big distraction, weightlifting, evolved into something even more consuming than Little 5 training.

I started a heavy workout regimen a few weeks after the ROTC Gala. If I was going to be in the reserves, I wanted to be the best, and to me, that meant the best physical shape possible. Fitness had already been a major part of my life during the previous three years of college, so going harder with it seemed like a reasonable next step. If the army stuff didn't work out, maybe I could at least become a personal trainer in the distant future.

An exercise program for every day was established; I had to work on my abs one day, my biceps and back the next, and so on. It wasn't the lifting itself that excited me, or even the gains in strength—although they were a nice bonus—but the other benefits. I quickly found that it made me happy to have a routine and be consistent for the first time since high school. It also made me happy to see the changes in my body—something I felt I could control. I wanted the bodybuilder physique. I had to appear powerful and fit. I grew obsessed with looking at myself in the mirror. I went home from my sessions with a sense of satisfaction, forgetting the larger dissatisfaction that lingered at the edges of my awareness.

Guiding me in my quest for physical perfection was Greg Nyland, an excellent friend and coach. Although his methods were unorthodox to others, our cussing and banter worked for us. "Yo, bro, you're acting like a bitch. Get that last rep up," he'd say. "Hey dickbag, just use the barbell. You can't handle plates," I'd reply. We did our best not to make noise in front of the other lifters, but we were borderline rude and obnoxious in our efforts to entertain each other.

Everyone I knew at the gym took multiple supplements. They encouraged me to do the same. When I was starting out, I saw their massive muscles and felt like I'd need to consume substances that were at least that hardcore if I wanted to emulate them. My bud Greg gave me a list of around ten to fifteen products he was using, and I ordered those products online without doing any research on them. My new exercise aids included BCAAs (branched chain amino acids), fish oil protein bases, various sets of random multivitamin packets, carb powder, and some ridiculously powerful pre-workout caffeinated substance. On top of all that were the testosterone boosters, none of which had received FDA approval. At twenty-two years old, I clearly didn't need any of this. But I believed it would give me that extra edge I needed to beat the competition.

All of these products were perfectly legal, giving the impression that they'd be beneficial at best, harmless at worst. What I didn't know was that some of my pre-workout supplements can keep a person up for twelve to sixteen hours at a time. If you take them at night, you will not sleep. The testosterone boosters were even more dangerous. Studies have shown that if you don't choose the correct ones, they can lead to increased anger and decreased self-control. Consuming a multitude of these substances and going beyond the recommended dosage of testosterone boosters led to a drastic change in my behavior toward others and the way I approached my relationships. While anger wasn't one of the side effects I experienced, lack of awareness was. I started to prioritize working out over my friends, my family members, and even the person who was supposed to be the love of my life.

Bev didn't approve of all the protein powder and chemicals I shoved into my body. She thought that I was acting primitive, that my personality was changing before her eyes. She called me a dirty caveman. And she wasn't alone. Several women told me they thought men who took all of these so-called nutrients were Neanderthals. I didn't care. The encouragement I received from my gym buddies who used the same substances outweighed what any woman might think.

Things came to a head one Saturday in late November. Bev showed up at my apartment when I was at the gym, having completely forgotten we were supposed to watch a movie together that night. Damn, that's why my phone had been buzzing incessantly in my pocket for a good ten minutes. *Oh shit, what do I say? Should I call her back right away or do this last set in front of the barbell rack first?*

I exited the back door of our campus gym and located a tranquil spot to call her, trying to think of an excuse for not being there. The guy I'd been working out with walked out right as she picked up the phone. I had Bev on speaker (I hate pressing the phone against my cheek) and didn't think to take her off.

"Dude! You slackin'?" my bud yelled. "Is this your way of pussying out of the last set?"

Bev heard all of it. "I see where your priorities are," she said calmly, and hung up on me.

Instead of rushing home to remedy the damage as quickly as possible, I looked at my friend and laughed. "Fuck her, dude, you can get a new chick anytime," he said.

Thirty minutes later, I came home to find a note on my door: "Fuck you, that's the last time I put up with your shit."

My heart didn't sink the way it had at the ROTC Gala. I just shrugged. I'd been hurt, so why shouldn't the people around me feel what I felt? The substances I was taking had altered my personality to the point where relationships no longer mattered. The only things I cared about were my personal progress and my distractions.

I became obsessed with the notion of getting bigger and stronger. By December, I could not go a single day without a pump. My competitive nature—and my need to be successful at something—drove me to not simply aim for self-improvement but to become the strongest person in the gym.

At some point post-breakup with Bev, I realized that I'd grown dependent on the substances I was using to achieve that goal. I couldn't function without consuming a variety of pre- and post workout drugs. The caffeine kept me energized and ready to go every second of the day. Testosterone helped me increase my gains at the gym. If I abstained from caffeine, testosterone, and BCAAs, I would feel dizzy and vomit. I felt like I was hooked on the protein and carb powder as well, even though they didn't affect me physically. So I was aware of the problem. I just didn't want to think of it as a problem. Any friend who questioned my intake of these drugs would've immediately been kicked out of my life, although no one ever pursued that route.

My addiction to workouts and workout aids, which grew worse by the day, led to an additional issue: sleep deprivation. Back in November, I'd been getting a good six to eight hours of sleep, so I still felt like a tank every morning when I woke up. As weightlifting consumed more of my time and the stimulants kept me going, my waking hours increased dramatically. It didn't help that 10:00 p.m. was "look at me hour." Many students didn't get out of class until later in the afternoon, and after that they would eat dinner and study. By the time the busier ones got done with their coursework, it would be around 9:00 or 10:00, and that's when they'd hit the gym. This was the time most people would approach me and congratulate me on my progress, motivating me further to be there until 11:00 or later.

But sleep no longer mattered to me. Recovery didn't matter either as long as I looked like I was successful. And I did. Every time I went in to lift, someone would ask me for advice. I didn't know jack shit about the specifics of fitness techniques, but I was muscular, so they figured I was an expert. Someone to look up to.

That's all I cared about.

9 SLEEP-DEPRIVATION SPIRAL

WHEN YOU COMBINE an enormous ego with a need to succeed in everything you do while taking on an abundance of tasks, the amount of time you have for each task dwindles rapidly. Unfortunately, hard work, a positive attitude, and inspirational videos will only get you so far when you only have twenty-four hours in a day. If it takes you five hours for homework, three for workouts, six for ROTC job stuff, three for meal prepping, one for walking to and from classes, and four for the party, you have two hours left.

Oh, but you decided to say yes to your neighbor when they asked you to move some furniture they're getting rid of into a loading truck. And then you say yes to one of your many flings. And then you . . . well, you are out of time, and you still have to shower, get your laundry clean, and do dishes.

The only reason you've even been able to get this much done is that the stimulants you're on have dramatically increased your number of waking hours. Working through the night seems like a good strategy that will enable you to catch up eventually.

The problem is, nobody should go even one day without sleep. Chronic sleep deprivation can make you more vulnerable to depression. It can also affect your mood, memory, and physical health in many surprising ways, all of which are unpleasant.

In my quest to take on all challenges, I managed to go for eight to twelve weeks without more than a few hours of sporadic, poor-quality sleep per day. Three months is all it took to go from sane to incredibly discombobulated.

DAY 1 AFTER NO SLEEP

It's late November or early December, a few weeks after starting my grueling workout regimen and training for the Little 500. In addition to Little 5 training and lifting, I have to manage schoolwork, ROTC assignments, and everything else that I've said yes to. I don't have the time I truly need for class anymore. This is going to be tough. Should I start skipping certain classes on certain days of the week to prioritize lifting? Loading up on coffee is the only option, I guess. I won't make it through the day without a high level of caffeine to keep me awake.

I've been taking a 300-level international studies class that meets three times a week. If I don't get at least a C+, I'll have to retake it next year, which means my ROTC scholarship will be taken from me and my dreams will go poof. We're asked multiple questions in every class, and maintaining at least a C+ requires a high level of participation and involvement.

In the middle of class, the professor asks, "Jacques, what are your thoughts on the walls being built and established on the Israeli–Palestinian border?"

My head hits the desk like a cracking coconut. Jolted out of my daydreams, I pulsate forward and respond with "Crackers." Yeah something is definitely wrong. My brain speaks to me:- *Dude, you're out of your gourd, bro.*

I get back to my apartment an hour and a half later and attempt to lie down so I can get an hour of sleep before my next class. It's 3:00. As soon as my head hits the pillow, my phone rings. A fraternity brother asks me to help him move several Little 500 bikes from the main room at our party complex and air up the tires for training later that night. No rest for me.

I attend my next class at 4:00, get done at 5:30, and walk home again. Immediately I get a text asking for help with logistical paperwork at the ROTC Department building regarding math and boring stuff. This lasts till 9:00 p.m. It's Monday, and already the week is off to a busy start.

But of course, I need to get my weightlifting in. At 10:00 I unwind at home for twenty minutes, then load up on supplements for a ninety-minute session. At a quarter to midnight, I still have four hours of homework to do for tomorrow's classes, which I procrastinated on until today. Using the public computers at the student library is easier than pulling out my laptop, which is on its last legs, so off to the library I go.

DAY 2 OF LITTLE TO NO SLEEP

It's 5:00 a.m. I'm finally done with my schoolwork. Suddenly I freak out, realizing I haven't looked at my phone since 10:00 p.m. Practice for the Little 500 is whenever our crew can make time to meet up and ride together, and sure enough, I missed it last night. I text our group, saying I'll make up for it by training this morning before school. I rush back to the complex, grab my bike, set off on a two-hour ride, and go back home to shower.

I'm still running on the pre-workout from the night before, but barely. I load up on pre-workout again, head to campus at 8:30, spend the entire class zoned out, and finish around 11:00 a.m. My surroundings are starting to get noticeably blurry. This isn't good, today is going to be useless, but going to bed isn't an option right now. I'll just catch up on sleep tonight.

My coordination, thoughts, and vision shift and pulsate slightly throughout the day. But I'm still walking and talking normally, fooling people around me into believing I'm totally in control of my thoughts. The day flies by quickly. Before I know it, it's 10:00 p.m. again. I haven't done my homework yet, and I've started to fall behind on my work. Three cups of coffee, one workout, and three hours of meal prepping later, my body and brain scream at me that we're going further down the rabbit hole, but... *Crap, it's 3:00 a.m. and I have to go to ROTC training in two hours.* I can't keep up. What am I going to do?

DAY 3

ROTC training is a one-hour blunder of a performance. My pride is crushed. I used to be one of the highest scorers on the physical fitness test. I did terribly on it this morning. Wednesday isn't looking so hot right now.

My mind is barely running at this point. It's time for three more cups of coffee and a dash of pre-workout to make it through the next twelve hours, hopefully.

By the end of the day, everything is spinning around me, I have a headache the size of Mars, and somehow I'm still functioning. I am not planning my time wisely. If I don't do something about my schedule, get organized, and get it in check now, this will spiral out of control. But I can't organize my thoughts in a way that enables me to do anything with this realization. It's like being high and trying to juggle three tennis balls upside down while composing a symphony.

This is the moment when I start losing my ability to process information from the outside world. I'm functioning at 50 percent or less.

DAY 6

It's Saturday, I haven't had a good sleep in what seems like an eternity, and I haven't consumed coffee for two days because I haven't had time to grab it or prep it. Despite both of these things, I feel as though I've gotten a second wind. I attempt a technique I learned in ROTC where you place your tongue on the roof of your mouth and shift it. It sounds weird, but constantly tickling the top of your mouth with your tongue will wake you up no matter what. Through pure determination, I stay up and complete almost all my work for ROTC, school, and my workout regimen. At 1:00 in the afternoon, I finally lie down.

I wake up to an obnoxious number of group texts vibrating through my phone. I missed Little 500 training at 2:00 p.m. I yell loudly and drag my feet out of bed. *That's it! That's enough.*

Right as I put on my bike clothes, I get a notification on my phone from one of my professors: there's a paper due on the Monday after next. I run the math in my head and realize there is nowhere near enough time to complete everything I need to do by then. Everything is crumbling around me. I'm losing focus, and I don't have a solution.

DAY 20, OR IS IT DAY 22?

With a great deal of effort, I've managed to scrounge an hour or two out of every other day to get sleep. It's not enough. My surroundings go from fuzzy to psychedelic. Literally psychedelic, as if I've taken DMT or shrooms. Colors around me are changing, and the kind of waves you'd see rippling in the horizon of a hot desert appear in the distance everywhere I walk. I am in a state of limbo where I'm almost incapable of distinguishing fiction from reality.

Was the conversation I had with him yesterday or today?

Was I supposed to turn in that paper yesterday?

Why are so many people staring at me by the bar downtown?

What the fuck, how did I get to the bar downtown? I don't remember walking here.

I am in a cosmic state of paranoia and vertigo. I am losing my damn mind. Or is this all just a dream from day 2? I don't know what's going on. I do know what's going on and I'm also completely confused. It is the most difficult, mind-bending experience one can describe. A euphoria-induced nightmare. I'm going to class one moment, partially aware of the tasks at hand; the next, I'm standing over my sink, staring into the abyss of an iron pan. This . . . this is insanity.

It's a beautiful thing.

This thought, "It's a beautiful thing," keeps entering my mind. It isn't really beautiful at all—but a sense of extreme relief washes over me in one fleeting moment as I finally realize I have no control over anything at all anymore. I sit hunched over a lit bedside candle and stare at it as the flame moves smoothly from left to right. *Whew, it's nice that I don't have to focus or concentrate on anything at all,* I tell myself. Beauty is danger and disorganization, and I'm okay with that.

My frame of mind, at this point, is an entirely new beast. A beast made up of every emotion a human can experience. Enjoyment, fear, and anxiety coexist simultaneously. I almost like the feeling. To me, it's the definition of working hard. You get what you put into your hard work. But none of that matters anymore. Beauty, danger, chaos, and hard work; it's all the same to me now.

MONTHS 2–3 (FOLLOWING CHRISTMAS BREAK)

I am capable of moving my hands and feet most of the time. I don't know how I'm awake right now. Has it been one week or one year since I last slept? Time does not exist. I don't exist. I go to school with half-pig, half-wolf people. *No, they're not hairy with snouts. That was just my imagination.* The pavement is winding up toward the sky. Have I missed class this week, or did I go and I don't remember? The wolf people cannot know I skipped class.

The most mind-boggling experience occurs after a two-foot-tall wooden lamp rises from the top of my ornately decorated bedside table. In front of the newly grown lamp is a seashell that wasn't there before.

"Hi there," I say to the seashell. "What's your name? Oh, that's fantastic. Would you like to come to class with me today? Oh, no? Well, what about tomorrow?"

The seashell leaps at me and threatens to bite me if I tell anyone I plan on bringing it to class. "My name's Tom the wily snapper, bitch—don't you forget it."

A seashell just threatened my life.

No way am I going to tell anyone that this occurred, not even my family. Even I know it sounds nuts. When a figment of my imagination says it's going to bite me and I'm not on any drugs, I know I have to sleep.

SATURDAY, FEBRUARY 14, 2015

I visit my mom and stepdad with a friend. We play with the dogs, eat some late lunch, and talk about graduation. My friend is graduating in May, and she asks me if I've ordered my cap and gown. This (according to my mom) is when I begin to act different. Soon we're all distracted once again by my family's new puppy. When asked again if I'm prepared for graduation, I tell her that all is under control. Little does she know that nothing is under control, including myself! (In fact, I don't remember this day at all. My mom had to fill in the details for me.)

FEBRUARY 17

At 3:00 a.m. I fall asleep. I wake up at 9:00 to find dozens of missed calls and text messages. I've missed ROTC training.

Having finally gotten six hours of uninterrupted sleep, my perception of what has occurred over the last couple of months is slightly clearer. I've fallen behind in everything—my work, workouts, Little 500 training, and the forty-page assignment that's due in less than twenty days. There is no way to catch up or make up for everything I've missed. I'm plunged into a state of confusion, stress, depression, and panic. I don't know what to do.

Ignoring all the calls and text messages, I bust open my laptop. Reports across the board in my gradebook online show C– or worse. Every one of my project assignments for ROTC is late. Gnats are buzzing around food that's been sitting out in my kitchen for God knows how long. Have I even eaten at all in weeks? What happened?

This moment is the breaking point. I don't know what to do. I'm screwed.

10 EXIT STRATEGY

BY THE END of the evening on February 17, I was in meltdown mode. It was a DEFCON 1 situation. *If only I had done this or that,* I thought over and over again, *I wouldn't be in the position I am in now.* An aura of hopelessness surrounded me, and I couldn't rid myself of it even if I tried.

The only thing I could think to do was drown all my fears in booze. Moonshine would do the trick. Not the number one plan I could have come up with, but I was incapable of processing anything at this point. I saw no reasonable alternatives, no way out. Whatever my solution would be, it'd have to wait. I might as well fail on my own terms. A drunken slugfest ensued from about 9:00 p.m. until who knows when in the morning. Clusters of disorganized thoughts haunted me as I fell into a stupor.

In the morning, extremely hungover, I attempted to reprocess the facts. I was going to drop out in my last semester of college. I was going to have to pay back tens of thousands of dollars in scholarship money. I was going to disappoint my Little 500 team.

My lieutenant colonel was already very disappointed in me for failing to turn in my assignment yesterday.

Looking back now, I wish I'd known how to talk to someone else about all of this when I hit bottom—or, better yet, when I started descending into psychedelic confusion. But my beliefs about what it meant to be a man drove me to do literally everything on my own. Fuck everyone else. Approaching anybody for help felt weak.

With no way out and (I believed) nowhere to turn, I could reach only one conclusion: *I have to give up.* I'm going to give up on my schoolwork. I'm going to quit going to the gym. I'm going to do nothing! Nothing matters now. Committing to this path of destruction the same way I'd committed myself to everything else, I considered the two options left to me at this point:

1. Suck it up, bite the bullet, and pay the consequences for my actions
2. Take my own life

Debating these options took the better part of what was left of the morning on February 18, 2015—which at this point was thirty minutes. Yeah, in less than thirty minutes, I decided whether I would live with my mistakes and attempt to correct them or end it all that day.

The first two minutes of pondering felt like two hours. I could only think of snow. I imagined snow falling in front of my face and landing on my nose and cheeks. I tilted my face toward the ceiling and envisioned a winter wonderland, relaxing just a little for the first time in months. I walked to the window next to the apartment entrance and stared out at the snow on the street with an empty gaze. *I don't have to think. For just one moment, I want to be blank.*

Fifteen minutes in, snowfall had exited my mind and was shifting to something grander. I imagined everyone I knew standing around me at my funeral. *How many people are there? Who will be the first to cry? Is anyone laughing? Who's the first to show up?* The questions went on and on as I imagined looking down at the casket from high above. Everyone surrounded the casket. They didn't notice me floating above them.

At around twenty-nine minutes in, I refocused on the decision at hand. Was it easier to die, or would I atone for my lack of prioritization?

It was clear now. I would end it all before allowing my humiliation to become known to those around me. I refused to care what family, friends, and others would think of my solution, although I was curious as to what tales people would tell of me. Would I be that campfire story a forty-year-old told his college buds? *"Hey, remember Jacques? It's crazy. It's been twenty years since he killed himself. I hope his family is doing all right."* Then I snapped out of it. It was over. I'd lost.

Death doesn't scare me, I repeated to myself. *I'm not afraid to die. This will be quick and easy.* I had search engines at my fingertips to figure out how to do it effectively.

Three options came to mind. I could overdose. I could slit my wrist—that sounded easy and doable. Or I could blow my head off—that would be quick. Having had some sporadic sleep in the previous days, I convinced myself that I was clear minded enough to pull this off and (just barely) coherent enough to drive.

My next thought: *Let's weigh the pros and cons of each option and figure out the details.*

Sitting in my apartment, I took out my phone and looked up the best drugs to overdose on. I considered heroin for a short while. Plenty of people used it downtown in our homeless community. I could buy twice the dose needed for a high and OD quite easily. But there was no way to get separate needles from a vendor that day, and if I survived my attempt, I didn't want to contract HIV. On to the next idea.

If I took a ridiculous number of over-the-counter painkillers, it might stop my heart. But too many would cause me to throw it up, meaning I'd have to start over with a new batch, and too little would give my kidneys and liver a fighting chance of metabolizing it. I wanted to be comfortable in my designated final moments and not have to shop again for meds if overdosing failed the first time. I'd add pills to the shopping list and look for backup options in case it didn't work.

With that in mind, which blade was the best for slitting wrists? A Bushman knife was far too large; it might get messy if I tried to use it to cut clean along my veins. I needed something small, but not too small. Razors would just fall out of my right hand from all the shaking I imagined I'd be doing. I needed to get a pocketknife or straight blade, carbon-steel tipped to be efficient. Stainless steel wasn't necessary because I didn't need to worry about rust; the knife only had to last one day. So, a carbon-steel-infused sharpened blade. Backup option two was set.

What could I blow my head off with if the first two methods failed? Many people survived gunshot wounds to the head from self-inflicted attempts when they used a handgun or semiautomatic rifle. I figured a shotgun with one shell would kill me effectively, tearing open the back of my skull, with no chance of leaving me paralyzed or a mindless vegetable.

What next? *Let's make sure these items are available locally.* There happened to be an excellent outdoor sporting goods store less than four miles from my apartment. I could grab the knife and shotgun in one visit. A pharmacy was on the way, so I would go there first and pick up the painkillers.

That was it. I had a plan.

• • • • • • •

After stopping at the pharmacy, I went to the sporting-goods place, put on my best poker face, and asked for a pack of 12-gauge shells. The clerk behind the counter stared at me intensely.

Why is she staring at me? I thought. *Is there a requirement that I look happy when buying a gun to kill myself?*

I had no prior record—just a simple drinking citation from my first semester—so passing the background check was no problem. Walking out of the store with the shotgun, I felt like I'd forgotten something. Oh! The knife! Whatever, I'd get one if I needed it later. I wasn't going back in there. I just needed to get this over with. I placed the shotgun and the pain reliever bottle on my back seat and covered them with a tan towel so no one would see them when I returned to my apartment.

Which brought me to the question of location. Should I do this in my apartment? No, too many people around, some of whom I knew. They'd hear me if I had to resort to the gun. Plus, a fraternity brother had been knocking on my door all morning, asking if I was in there. I needed to go to some other town where nobody recognized me. Somehow, the thought of it taking an extra twelve to twenty-four hours for my parents, other family members, and friends to find out about my death made it easier. If the painkillers worked, no one would hear me pass away, so any signs of my dying would remain hidden within the walls of some building until it was far too late for anyone to try to save me.

What building, though, and where? It could be a motel. I could turn on the bath, and the loud running water would cover any noise I made, ensuring that it'd take longer for people to find my body.

I couldn't forget to gas up before I went. I needed to make sure I had enough to make it to whatever middle-of-nowhere town I found.

Yeah, that's it. I got it now, I told myself. *I'm going anywhere but here.* I'd just hop on the highway, traveling in any direction, and eventually I'd pass by a motel two to three hours from home. I'd stop there, rent a room for the night, and set everything up. I just needed to remember to stop somewhere on the way out of town and get a knife first. I might have to settle for whatever the store had.

I drove back to my apartment building and parked on the opposite side of the street, looking around to see if anyone who knew me saw me pull up. I walked back in, checked everything, and made sure no one had left a note at my door. And no, I didn't leave a suicide note or anything like that. When the idea of doing so occurred to me, I shrugged it off. *This is it. I don't care what people think of my last thoughts. They're mine and mine alone to have.* I genuinely felt no need to write an emotional explanation of why I'd decided to end my life.

Did I have any consideration for how others would feel after my passing? No, I didn't. With no way out of the labyrinth, I was on a mission, and my type-A personality wouldn't let anything get in the way. There was nothing left to think over. I'd made up my mind. Time to go—no looking back.

11
VOYAGE TO THE UNKNOWN

AN EERILY UNFAMILIAR emotion that I hadn't felt since I was incredibly young—fear—presented itself. As I walked out to my car to begin my journey to the afterlife, fear crept into all of my pores and manifested in the form of goosebumps and sweats. Time slowed to a crawl. In my highly sleep-deprived state, opening the car door took ten seconds and felt like an hour. Sitting in the car seat took another ten-second hour.

I inserted a CD that would help put me in the right frame to execute my plan. *Ring of Fire* by Johnny Cash made more sense to me in that moment than anything else I was experiencing. It helped calm my nerves and set the tone perfectly. With the ignition started and my goals aligned with the mood music, I began my drive.

This part was blurry. A miniature blackout occurred. I didn't recognize my surroundings throughout the entire . . . who knows, two, four, six hours of driving? All I could do was stare into the abyss of the windshield. Trees passing on my right and left appeared as convoluted, wavy figures as the sky spit icy snow. I felt as if nature was watching me.

Two voices in the back of my mind kept telling me what to do. One said, "No, you still have a choice. You can turn around now and go back. I'm sure you can find your way back. Right?" The other said, "Yes, you've come this far, you've made your choice clear, now man up and complete it. Don't baby out of it now." The ongoing battle overwhelmed my senses. *This is crazy! But it's not that crazy. I mean, I don't have a choice, correct?*

My Johnny Cash CD started over at track 1, snapping me back to reality. The trees that had been moving like a mirage grew still as I crested the ridge of an industrial-looking area. *Did I just drive to a city?* I had no idea how long I'd been on the road, but it hadn't gotten dark yet.

In the meantime, my old iPhone's battery was low. I had no GPS or maps in my car, so the phone was my only option for finding a motel. I needed to charge it before it died on me.

I spotted a high-rise hotel down the valley and stopped there, gathering my thoughts for the hundredth time. On the other side of a large window stood an older woman with prominent wrinkles and braids running down the left side of her face. It looked like maybe a young granddaughter had tried to do her hair and butchered the job, but she kept the lopsided braids anyway out of love for her and her effort. The woman stared through the window into my car, watching me.

Or, maybe she wasn't watching me so much as just doing her job at the front desk. When your state of mind has deteriorated to the point where pursuing death feels like a good idea, it seems as though everyone around you is observing you. You think they know what you're up to, even if they don't.

I opened the front door of my car slowly, got out, and walked in. The woman greeted me at the front desk and asked if I needed anything. I asked her if I could borrow an outlet for half an hour to charge my phone.

Of course, I could've just gotten a room here. Money didn't matter to me anymore. But this wasn't the place. My journey couldn't end in a fancy hotel. I preferred the classic romantic gesture of ending it in a droopy motel, like in the movies. It would better suit my situation.

And I needed every excuse I could muster not to stop just yet.

She looked at me, pretending not to. Or was I just paranoid, overanalyzing every situation, every interaction? Now for sure she thought something strange was going on because I was reacting to her reacting. Maybe this stranger felt the same way I do. Why did I feel like I was connecting more with her than anyone I'd ever known? The thought *This could be the last person I ever see* played repeatedly in my head. I gave her my largest, fakest, smile.

"Do I need to call somebody?" she said. "Are you feeling okay?"

"No, I'm perfectly fine."

I clearly wasn't. If I'd chosen to tell her the truth, the day could have gone a completely different direction. But I felt as if I were being bothersome. I didn't want to annoy her with an explanation, even if it meant saving my own life and the mental well-being of others in my circle. I was genuinely worried about this cute old lady and how this small conversation would impact her. If she was the last person I ever talked to, at least I could smile at her and go out on a good note.

Thirty minutes passed. After retrieving my phone, I headed back to my car, pulled up Maps, and found a motel only five minutes away. I could've easily gotten there without the battery running out.

The motel parking lot was covered with snow, as if it hadn't been shoveled all week. A scraggly-looking older man sat behind the clerk's table in a small reception room, and I scrutinized him, taking in every detail. He looked like he survived on a diet of cornflakes and drama. The belly button piercing that poked out of the bottom of his shirt told me everything I thought I needed to know about his fitness level—Jenny Craig was no match for this man's appetite. There's no way he enjoyed his job. What kind of life did he have outside of this establishment? I assumed he went home every night, yelled at his wife, retreated to a corner of his trailer home, and put himself to sleep with alcohol. Was his situation any better than mine? Was he any happier than me? More importantly, was he willing to kill himself like I was?

Yeah, my mean, judgmental college attitude carried over even into my supposed final hours on this planet. Comparing my life to that of other unfortunates around me felt like the only solace I could obtain in my all-is-lost mindset.

I walked up to the desk. "Hi sir, how much is a room?"

He grumbled loudly. "This one is thirty-four bucks. Hey! And don't run the water for more than a few minutes." He handed me a key and collected $34.56.

I had one more question—the question that had been bugging me all day. "Hey, what city am I in?"

He gave me a look of confusion. "Are you messing with me, boy? You're in Florence, Kentucky."

Okay, good. I was far enough away from home!

The room was as I expected: Dirty, in shambles, and falling apart at the floorboards and seams. A mosh pit of mites. I assessed my surroundings. *Where can I place the shotgun? Or should I just leave it in my car under the blanket?* Another idea popped into my head: What about carbon monoxide poisoning? No, I didn't have enough time to plan it out. I should have thought of that before I left.

Over-the-counter painkillers were left on the dusty bedside table with the shotgun leaning against a dusty chair beside it. What were the next steps?

Time passed quickly, and the dim lights within the room grew inexplicably bright. *Is this still a dream, or am I really doing this? Am I really this close to literally pulling the trigger on my decision?*

The only thing missing was a knife. I'd kept forgetting to purchase one before. An immediate sense of relief poured over me. Procuring this final item gave me an excuse to put off killing myself for at least another hour.

I found another sporting store near the motel, and they had the exact knife I was looking for. Everyone around me in the check-out line could tell something was off, though—I was sure of it. *Is there any reason no one is stopping me from doing this?*

I told myself that they wouldn't step in because our culture condemns speaking truthfully in such situations—another lame excuse I came up with to avoid taking responsibility for my own actions. In retrospect, my poker face ensured that no one had a clue as to what I was thinking.

Knife in hand, I realized that it was going to be extremely difficult to pull this off if I wasn't decently inebriated. A six-pack of beer would do the job.

Okay, why didn't I think of all of this before I left? Did I rush my decision? Is all of this a terrible, terrible dream? I can still stop this! Only I have the power to do it.

I pushed past my doubts and hit a liquor store at the corner of the sporting-goods market before walking back to my car. Hopefully six beers with 7.5 percent alcohol content would be enough to enable me to move forward.

Driving back to the motel, I did everything I could to put off my demise, slowing down to look at statues and bushes and taking detours that made the trip thirty minutes instead of ten. The man at the front desk was still there when I got back. We briefly made eye contact before I slowly creaked my door open and entered. Time to unpack the knife and beer. Enough stalling. The buildup was tearing me apart.

I removed the painkillers from two identical packages, then started on the beers. The entire six-pack was gone in thirty minutes. Still alert and aware of my surroundings, I consumed dozens of pills in twenty seconds. I got halfway through downing a dozen more before puking everything up.

Well, that failed.

Time to move on to option 2. The sharp blade of my newly acquired knife was slowly drawn from its sheath, and my feet dragged my body over to the mirror. With the knife in my hand, I looked down at my left wrist and back up at myself, repeating this process incessantly over the next twenty minutes.

What I needed was warm bathwater. Without that, it would be impossible to cut cleanly through my wrist and up through my forearm. I turned the faucet all the way to the right, and hot water pooled into the tub. According to what I found online, this would be quick, easy, and minimally painful. Not that pain was going to be an issue—I'd had kidney stones before, and this couldn't be any worse. With the water filled to the brim of the tub, I begin taking off my clothes.

Someone knocked.

"Sir! Sir, can you come to the door?"

What the hell. What was this about?

I creaked open the door in the same slow, drawn-out manner as I had when I last entered. It was the man from the front desk.

"Hey, so I just wanted to check," he said as snowflakes filled the entryway. "I heard the water running for quite a long time, and the water here gets expensive. Just make sure you finish as quick as you can."

This was my chance! My final opportunity to reach out for help before taking my life. Why wasn't he stopping me? Did he not see the shotgun by the chair? I looked back; the firearm was fairly well concealed with my coat hanging next to it, so maybe he didn't. Or did he?

A bleak look crossed the man's face as he passed a glance behind me. He knew. I'd been discovered. Now he could call the cops and report to them what he saw. Or he could just stop me right here, right now.

"Okay," I said. That one word was all I could muster.

He turned around and walked away. *No . . . I've lost my chance.*

Now all I could do was drag myself back to the tub before the water got cold and do this quickly. My patience had worn thin. I didn't even bother to take my clothes off. I just dipped my forearm in there and got it over with.

Well, I tried to get it over with. Turned out every movie and every Reddit post was wrong. Cutting myself *fuckin' hurt.* I only managed to make it two millimeters across my wrist. I stuffed my mouth with my socks so no one would hear the screaming and yelling coming from my room. *Dear God, how can anyone do this? I've got to stop right now. I can't go through with it, at least not this way. Nuh-uh.*

I felt deflated. I thought I had planned this so well. This was all an idiotic idea. "Fuuuuccckkk!"

The shotgun was the only option I had left. I had to make it count.

Loading the shotgun, unlike previous steps I'd attempted, went smoothly and quickly due to my military experience. I tilted the shotgun toward my face and stared down the barrel into the deepest void that had ever existed. It was pitch black, and I couldn't see the bottom.

All I had to do is take the safety off and pull the trigger. Painless and quick. Nothing compared to the knife.

I switched off the safety, and my index finger inched down toward the outside of the trigger guard. I twitched uncontrollably. Sweat covered my palms. The shotgun slipped out of my hands, and I caught it midair before the butt of the rifle touched the ground and discharged a shell. That was close.

Over the course of an hour, I put the barrel in my mouth and pulled it back out, again and again. I lost what felt like ten pounds of sweat. I didn't pull the trigger. I couldn't.

The shotgun reclaimed its rightful place at the dusty bedside table.

I was out of options, and the day was almost gone. I needed to do something. It didn't matter what.

Well, there was one other way to make this happen. I could fire a shell into the air, throw the safety on, jam the gun, and wait for the police to arrive. Then I'd point it somewhere above their heads, and they'd have no choice but to shoot me.

I tried so, so hard with all my remaining willpower to think of an alternative. The police didn't deserve to be put in this position. Taking a man's life isn't easy, and I was about to force them to do it.

But no other option came to me.

I walked into the blistering snow and headed to the back of my car, hoping no shells would penetrate further than my vehicle when the police opened fire. I held the shotgun firmly to my shoulder and fired two shells.

The police arrived in less than five minutes.

"Put it down!"

"Place it on the ground!"

"Throw it down!"

My mind went blank, not able to decipher all the screaming and yelling, until I heard one of them say, "Please, I don't want to do this! Please!"

They *knew*. They knew I wanted to kill myself.

But before I could fully process that thought—*bang*.

12
NOWHERE IS HERE

NUMEROUS BANGS AND pops followed the first shot, and my body fell to the ground like a rag doll, my face planting against the rock-hard snow. A void appeared before my eyes—a black hole leading to nowhere. My eyes shut, and I felt myself fade into oblivion. After everything that had happened, it was over. No more sadness or fear. I could finally rest.

I just hoped the ridiculously high level of pain would dissipate soon.

While I couldn't see anything, I was just conscious enough to hear the many officers who surrounded me. One performed lifesaving procedures while my blood pooled in the snow. I woke up briefly to see a tourniquet being wrapped around my left arm. The blood encasing my body helped keep me warm.

This isn't good, and the pain isn't going away. This isn't good, and the pain isn't going away. I wanted to scream, but my mind couldn't translate my thoughts into speech and, in any case, both of my lungs had been penetrated, making it impossible to produce sounds.

I'm not dead! What just happened? Why am I not dead?

"Give me the wrap!"

"Bring it now!"

"Why did you do this?" one of the officers yelled.

"Bring it here now!" was the last thing I heard before passing out.

My eyes blinked open again. I was in an ambulance, facing multiple syringes adjacent to my head. Tubes hung from every crevice of my body. My shirt was torn off, revealing my stomach—which had been blown wide open. I desperately mumbled whatever I could in an attempt figure out what was going on.

A paramedic met my eyes. "Okay, he's still with us."

Did I die, or am I still here? There's no way I survived this. As everything went black for the second time, I thought, *Hopefully this is permanent.*

It wasn't. My eyes opened to an extremely bright light that shone in an otherwise eerily dark room. I didn't believe in heaven—I thought we just turned to dust when we died—but I didn't have another explanation for the light, and it was hard to believe that I'd really made it all the way to a hospital without dying.

As these thoughts swirled around in my mind, I became aware of the sounds around me. A lot of talking, with commands from various individuals being thrown in every direction. The light moved away from me.

No, come back! I wanted to scream the words, but as before, they didn't escape my mouth. *If it's real, then I guess I didn't get in.* I'd been rejected by God. Maybe. I kept hoping all of this was just an awful dream. I would learn later that my heart had completely stopped, and I'd already died twice for more than two minutes.

As the lamp light in the surgery room faded, I counted at least fifteen surgeons and nurses attending to my wounds. "Get the fib!" I heard while drifting in and out of consciousness. "We're going to need it!"

Euphoria set in again slowly. Now the entire room was filled with lights. The crowd had dissipated, and all that remained were two nurses, each of whom appeared to have a specific job pertaining to my well-being. My thoughts became more coherent.

I'm still here?

I shouldn't have attempted to kill myself. I was still in extreme pain, and it wasn't going away. In fact, it had gotten much, much worse. No amount of morphine or Dilaudid would help. Why did I choose to do this?

What is happening?

My mind clung to the hope that this was a dream. I kept trying to convince myself that none of it was real.

The two nurses began talking with each other as I observed the tubes and syringes that had been stuck inside of me. Blood filled the tubes quickly, disappeared, and reappeared. The nurses finished their tasks and headed for the door. But before they left, they looked at me and stared back at each other.

"How do you want to kill him?" the blond female nurse said.

"Let's start with the bones," said the tall male nurse. "Let's break every one of them. He should survive that. Then we can grab bags of sand from the basement and fill his veins with sand. But we want to make sure he doesn't die quickly."

"Great idea! He deserves to suffer for what he did," the blond nurse proclaimed. "You know what we can do with the fingernails, right?"

"You mean after we chop his fingers off and feed them to Harold? He'll just spit the fingernails out. Then we can collect them and add them to our necklace," the tall nurse said. "His ribs are still intact. Let's take them out one by one, and we can sword fight with them."

"But then he's not going to have a stable stomach."

"That won't be an issue," the tall nurse said. "We'll just chop off the bottom part of his body and replace it with robot parts. He'll still be able to press buttons and call us if he needs us before we pour acid on his face and kill him."

All I could do throughout this terrifying exchange was make eye contact. I couldn't speak, and I couldn't quite figure out why. Rattling the straps that held me down was the only way to escape. I had to break them!

After the nurses left, an earsplitting shriek came from the hallway again. This was my chance. Frantically, I attempted to pull all the tubes out of my body and get off the bed. But I couldn't move.

Why am I stuck to the torture bed? The tubes can't be removed, so they must be holding me down. I'm in a damn cartel cannibal torture facility, not a hospital. Who or what the fuck is Harold?

A man with a melting face walked into the room. Harold. It had to be Harold. Shaking uncontrollably, I attempted to yell, "Take my fingers, but please don't kill me." But once again, no words came out.

How could a place like this exist? Most horror movies didn't approach this level of bloodcurdling creativity.

"Jacques, listen to me," Harold said, speaking with a woman's voice. "It's your mother." The man—Harold, my mother, whoever this was—left without eating my fingers. No one could be trusted!

The nurses reentered the room and immediately got to work on my ribs. One by one, they were sucked out of my torso and placed in a metal tray. Now I really couldn't move. If I'd had any chance of escape, it was gone now.

• • • • • • •

As you may have guessed, all of the horror-movie elements of my experience were a product of my imagination. More specifically, they were a product of narcotic-induced psychosis, also known as intensive-care-unit psychosis. I required a far higher level of pain medication than most patients due to the extent of my injuries. When an abundance of narcotics is introduced into a person's system while that person is on a ventilator, in a dimmed room, hooked up to IVs, and so on, it creates a sense of paranoia coupled with extreme hallucinations. Of course, I couldn't understand this at the time, and unfortunately, reducing the medication wasn't a viable option. What they were giving me wasn't even enough. So many parts of my body had been damaged that I was incapable of having pain meds delivered to portions of my legs and arms due to excessive blood loss and lack of adequate blood flow. So the living nightmares continued. There was no end to them, from my perspective, and no escape.

It took a long time to come down. For weeks, possibly months, I remained convinced that the nurses were trying to kill me, and I wasn't 100 percent sure that the events of my initial psychosis-induced dreamscape hadn't actually occurred. But about a week after hallucinating the removal of all my ribs, my perceptions started lining up with what was happening in the real world. That's when I truly came face to face with the consequences of my actions.

A nurse walked into the room with one of the trauma surgeons who saved my life. My eyes were closed, but I could hear them talking with my mother and stepfather.

"There are multiple gunshot wounds to the chest, left arm, right leg, right hip, abdomen, and groin areas," the surgeon said. "We'll try everything we can to save his life, but I'm not sure we can save the arm." A bacterial infection, I learned, was eating its way through my left forearm.

Although I didn't know it yet, I'd been placed on antidepressants pretty much immediately after my first lifesaving surgeries. The nurses and a forensic psychologist basically told me I had to be on them. It was a good idea. They likely put me in a better state of mind than I'd been in when I believed it was a good idea to force the police to kill me. But no antidepressant could shield me from the impact of this news. I was going to lose my arm!

Yet another new nurse walked into the room. My mind clearer now, I watched her assess me from my neck down to the bottoms of my feet. I looked at my body for the first time since the ambulance and wanted to throw up. My chest and abdomen were a puzzle of gaping wounds, tubes sprouting from everywhere. To the left of my navel sat a colostomy bag. Yeah, I'd messed up big time. There was no coming back from this.

Over the next few months, I had so many surgeries that I lost count. I was taken off the ventilator only to be put back on it numerous times. I moved in and out of different units within the trauma hospital. My body felt like a revolving door, with each new day bringing a new painful procedure. I had been shot twelve times. My abdomen, chest, liver, lungs, stomach, intestines, left arm, left leg, and groin all sustained traumas. I didn't know if I would ever be able to use my left arm again, walk, or be free of the colostomy bag. I had a belly full of skin grafts to hold my abdomen together because the original skin there was shredded or gone. My intestines and stomach were herniating—that is, bulging through an abnormal body opening—and the resulting lacerated tissue would also require skin grafts. The grafts would be taken from my right thigh, so even this area of my body that hadn't been riddled with bullets would be full of trauma and scarring.

13 VISITORS AND ADVOCATES

OF COURSE, I wasn't the only one dealing with the consequences of my actions. They took an unimaginable toll on everyone who rallied to support me.

My mother drove two hours, five to seven times a week, to see me. While I wasn't aware of it at the time, she wasn't just providing emotional support—she was the point person for all communication, advocating unceasingly for me and my future. Behind the scenes, she met with social workers, attorneys, Indiana University administrators and professors, ROTC, the police, and my physicians. She'd been a nurse, although she hadn't practiced for years, and she fought tooth and nail to make sure my left arm wasn't amputated. Though I would have many surgeries on it and months of occupational therapy, today I maintain almost full mobility of that arm. My mother's incessant chattering had irritated me more than just about anything else in this world when I was in high school, but her words and perseverance saved my limb, and quite possibly my life.

My father played a different role in my recovery. I'd never seen a man as quiet as he was when he entered my room. He seemed to banish all of his thoughts to a remote corner of his mind, only speaking when an important matter involving nurses or surgeons presented itself. It was strange seeing this robust, confident man stuck in his own head. But his actions said everything; he didn't have to speak. As unremarkable as it sounds, being there at my bedside was all I needed from him. Seemed like I ended up spending more time with him in this hospital than I had since the divorce.

My dad never asked why I didn't just come to him and ask for help, though I'm sure the question crossed his mind. After several visits, when he was finally able to articulate his thoughts, he said, "I spoke with you the day you tried to kill yourself, and I had no clue that you were feeling like this."

My stepfather, Mark, wasn't a big fan of visiting people in the hospital. He worked as a hospital administrator and preferred to get away from that setting during his off hours. But he came to see me often, and he voiced his support clearly when he did. "We'll figure this out," he said on many occasions. "Yeah, it was dumb, and there will be consequences, but I'm going to help," Most of my visiting family members talked about my emotions; Mark showed his love for me in a different way, talking about the problems I faced and proposing solutions in a way that was direct and to the point. I would trust the man to fight for me with his life. He worked himself half to death attempting to help me with my legal and medical issues.

Of all my family members, the one who was hit the hardest was Lucas, the seventeen-year-old brother I'd teased incessantly when I was a kid. He'd always seemed to possess a level of maturity far surpassing his chronological age. He never broke any rules and always did the right thing, maybe because he learned from the mistakes of all his older siblings. Every Friday after school, he drove several hours one way to visit me. He gave up high school athletics to be there for me.

Instead of asking me why I did it, he simply said, "I love you. You doing okay?" He sipped the coffee he brought with him every time he came, stared at it, and looked around the room. "You know I love you, right?" he kept repeating. In retrospect, I'm guessing that he said this to comfort himself, desperately struggling to hold himself together.

We had never been particularly close, mainly due to the difference in our ages, but I think he always wanted to be. For my suicide attempt to be what broke the ice and enabled us to develop a relationship is extremely saddening to me. I wonder now if he felt like he should have known how I was feeling, even though I'd intentionally kept it hidden from everyone. In any case, the ordeal was arguably one of the factors that drove him to pursue a career in medicine. He wanted to be a surgeon and save lives, especially after seeing how they saved my life.

After a few months passed, two very special people came to the hospital to visit me. One was a great friend of mine, Mare Bear, whom I had known since my freshman year. I'd considered her one of the guys; we hung out at frat parties together, and I gave her advice about whoever she was seeing. Mare was talkative, and her chatter in this new setting helped lighten the rather somber mood. I'm glad she did most of the talking—I would've broken down then and there if I had been able to get a single word in.

Then there was Dave, my best bud from college, who'd been in the ROTC program with me for the first few years.

"You idiot, why did you do that?" Dave said upon entering my room on a quiet afternoon. "You could have just told me you were feeling like this." Those were the first words out of his mouth, and damn, they sunk in quickly—I let out a laugh for the first time in months.

You may have noticed that I've described everyone else's words and actions during these visits except my own. The truth is, as I lay in my hospital bed throughout most of this journey, I felt blank. Emotionless. As each person attempted to communicate, I mostly muttered minimal responses to direct questions. Nothing mattered to me. This seemed as low as I could go. I couldn't tell if I was depressed or detached, but confronting the reality of my situation was the last thing I wanted to do. In the meantime, everyone around me was experiencing every emotion known to man, but no one wanted to show how much my suffering affected them. The last thing they wanted was for me to worry about them worrying.

14 LEGAL AND FINANCIAL TROUBLES

TWO WELL-DRESSED MEN with deep voices walked into my hospital room and introduced themselves. They reminded me a bit of the Men in Black, ready to leap into action at a moment's notice. But instead of doing battle with aliens, their job was to fight legal problems.

With my parents on both sides of the family sitting in the room with me, my new attorneys explained the situation calmly and clearly. I'd broken the law, they explained, but they were there to help.

"So, the prospects are not great," said Tony Garfield, the younger of the two. "Unfortunately, a firearm was involved."

Bill Schmidt, taller and much older, nodded. "The police will do everything they can to make you appear to be a criminal."

Apparently I had been charged with six counts of wanton endangerment—which took me by surprise, to say the least. I'd never thought of myself as a criminal. I'd tried to kill myself, and now I was apparently being punished for it on top of being severely injured. I didn't express my indignation, though. I was barely able to do more than mutter brief answers to their questions.

"We'll do what we can to minimize damages and corroborate with the detectives in confirming it was a suicide attempt," Tony continued. "This will help immensely."

They concluded that my best option was to take a plea deal for the few counts of wanton endangerment that involved endangering only myself. If I didn't accept that deal and the case went to trial, there was a fifty-fifty chance I would lose on every front. Instead of pleading, the prosecutors would attempt to add assault with a deadly weapon to the charges. That would most likely result in a life sentence.

Negotiations with the police and prosecutors' office began, and my attorneys fought tooth and nail to ensure that I didn't end up in a prison cell. While they toiled on my behalf, I felt completely crushed. All I could do for the next year was wait to find out what would happen to me—whether I'd spend the rest of my life rotting in prison, whether I'd eventually be able to walk or use my left arm again, whether my stomach could be fixed, whether my colostomy could be reversed, and whether anyone would ever look at me the same. The only thing I knew for sure was that I was a million dollars in debt. The pulsating fear that had lived in the back of my head since arriving at the hospital shifted its focus from hallucinations of torture to the legal repercussions of my actions. This was never going to end.

• • • • • • •

Many months after our first meeting, my attorneys entered my hospital room for the third or fourth time. They had a plan that would hopefully reduce my scary potential life sentence to a more moderate one. Bill took charge this time.

"So we discussed several options together," he said. "We think it would be wise if you were to meet with the detectives, one-on-one, and answer any questions they have." Based on their experience, speaking with them would show that I had nothing to hide. Refusing the meeting meant taking a chance on a court hearing.

Bill and Tony ran through some of the questions the detectives might ask: "What was your intent that night?" "Did you intend to harm yourself or others?" There was a strong possibility that they'd tell me, "We looked at your phone and know everything." Whatever their questions were, the way I answered would determine my fate. "When answering a question," Tony emphasized, "tell the truth. You have nothing to hide, so hide nothing!"

The lawyers exited, leaving me to my thoughts. But before I had too much time to obsess over the stakes of my impending interrogation, my mother entered the room. She had news of her own. Turns out that a tiny clause in my health insurance portfolio at the bottom of page three thousand four hundred and bull crap stated that it was within their rights to cancel my policy if I was hurt "in the process of committing a crime." In other words, they would not be paying for my hospitalization.

"Don't worry about the bills," she said, attempting to sugarcoat her announcement with the sweetest words she could muster. "We can switch you over to Medicaid or another health insurance company, and they'll cover it. I love you, and I don't want you to worry about any of it."

Mom took the reins, spending hours and hours on phone calls and letters back and forth to switch me to Medicaid. The bureaucracy involved was intense and painstakingly slow; it took her a month and a half to complete the process. Still, her efforts eased my mind a little, allowing me to hope I wouldn't be footing a ridiculously large medical bill—or, more accurately, bills, plural. Maybe I'd managed not to destroy at least one area of my life.

But two months later, I found out I owed millions of dollars to the hospital—sorry, hospitals, plural—for care incurred under my former insurance carrier. Every twenty-four hours I'd gone without coverage, I owed another $20,000 to $40,000. I would have to file bankruptcy.

Luckily, I had no assets to my name. I would be losing nothing, I guess, except for my pride, ego, use of limbs, and just about everything else that I believed had defined me as an individual.

And I'd thought I was depressed before.

15 INTERROGATION AND RUMINATION

"HI, I'M HARRY. This is my partner, Boxer. Good to meet you for the fifth time."

It had been two months since Tony and Bill had recommended that I speak with the detectives in charge of my case. You'd think that I'd feel prepared after all that time, but my primary emotion was confusion. I'd had the idea that these guys would storm in all gung ho, screaming at me about the terrible things I'd done. I didn't expect Harry's calm, friendly demeanor or his kind smile. I also couldn't tell if he was joking.

"What do you mean five times?"

"I assumed you probably wouldn't remember," Boxer said in a sterner tone.

"Well, the first night when you arrived at the hospital, we were the first officers to speak to you," Harry explained. "You said, 'Just let me die. I don't care anymore.'" What a great first impression I made on them, huh?

"This won't be where we're asking the questions," Harry said. "That'll be in the rec room. But we wanted to introduce ourselves and see if you needed anything before heading over." When I declined to make any requests, he continued. "So, we'll be asking a few questions so that we can get a clear idea of what happened that night. Just to make sure, is this all right with you?"

"Yes, sir," I responded quietly. In my mind, I had no choice but to obey.

For security reasons, they'd demanded that our meeting be held in a public forum like a cafeteria or breakroom. That meant shifting my broken body out of the hospital bed and migrating to a larger table down the hall so that I could speak with them.

A nurse helped me transfer out of my bed. *Here we go! Left foot first. Okay, now shuffle it very, very slowly to the right, aaannnd bingo!* The left foot had a sock on it. I repeated the procedure with my right foot. Great! That only took thirty minutes. Now for the hard part: lifting myself out of bed and hauling all of my body weight over to a wheelchair.

I rarely, if ever, needed to get up to pee or do anything else, so I'd had little opportunity to practice leaving the bed. To prepare myself for today, I'd mentally rehearsed this maneuver a thousand times over. *Okay, time to shine,* I told myself. *I can do this.*

Propelling my arms forward and holding onto the bed's grip bar with my good arm, I thrust myself up onto my right leg, trying not to put any weight on my injured left leg. This gave me a few seconds to pivot my feet into the chair before I collapsed. I failed the first attempt. *But I'm almost there,* I kept telling myself as pain surged up and down my body. I gave out a quick yelp and attempted for a second time to lift myself. Success! Pain consumed my legs and arms, then shifted to a new location as my ribs cracked.

It took me well over an hour to get from the hospital bed to a wheelchair and then to the table in the rec room, only fifty feet from my door. If this was a test to determine whether I was as damaged as I claimed, I guess I passed. Now, with my entire body aching, it was time to assume my role as the main antagonist in a TV cop drama. Boxer and Harry greeted me again at the entrance of the room as I wheeled myself over to a table. My attorneys sat to the left and right of me, observing.

"So, we have a few questions for you regarding the events and what occurred," Boxer said. "Can you tell us your motive for trying to harm an officer?"

Oh shit. I didn't expect that at all. It was obvious from my perspective that I'd been trying to kill myself—hurting anyone else was not my intent. But in retrospect, Boxer might've just been playing the role of "bad cop." With his aviator sunglasses, aura of authority, and muscle-toned body reminiscent of how my father looked to me when I was three, he was a natural for the part. It was clear that he read people very well, cutting through bullshit with a soldering knife. Harry, projecting a laid-back, friendly persona and wearing innocuous plaid clothes with a ridiculous number of pockets, gave more of a "good cop" vibe.

"Well, let me ask again," Boxer said before I could answer. "Were you attempting to hurt them?"

"No," I mumbled.

"Okay," he said more forcefully, "then why did you aim a gun at officers?"

"I didn't. I promise."

"I'm sorry, I couldn't hear you. Speak up," Boxer demanded.

"I'm sorry. It's just hard to speak," I said quietly.

Boxer settled down a little and sat back in his chair, dialing down his intensity to match my obvious nervousness.

"We found a long list of searches in your phone's search history that we confiscated," Harry said. "Can you explain to us why you looked up how to kill yourself dozens of times?" Weird question. A hundred searches must've made my intentions clear to them. "We just have to ask," he said as I attempted to lift my heavy head and mumble another reply. "I'm sorry. I know it's tough to answer."

Boxer kept staring at me with increasing severity throughout this line of questioning; he'd probably received advanced training on how to intimidate suspects with eye contact alone. Then he shifted his gaze from me to a spot on the floor to his right—and a tear welled up below his right eye. I may have been the only one to see it. I'm sure he hoped I didn't notice, as his job required that he remain composed at all times. That was the moment when the detectives went from being bad guys in my mind to ordinary people doing their jobs like everyone else. They were human, just like me.

After a few more questions and mumbled responses, Harry and Boxer took off, leaving me to my increasingly unpleasant thoughts.

My primary concerns up to this point had been about myself: Would I recover from my injuries? Pay off my debts? Avoid prison and lead anything resembling a normal life? Now I focused on the myriad ways my actions had affected others beyond my inner circle. Florence, Kentucky, had a high crime crate for such a small town. When I put police officers in a situation where they had to shoot me, I took away their ability to save other people who might have been in danger. Dealing with the aftermath diverted resources from their department that were desperately needed elsewhere. Why had I been so selfish?

With all the reports of police brutality in the news, now is a good time to make something abundantly clear: none of the officers involved in my case did anything wrong. In fact, they went above and beyond the call of duty, doing everything they could to save my life. And their service didn't end there. My mother, who worked with the police from day one, told me years later that she couldn't have gotten through the trauma of my attempt had it not been for the sincerity and professionalism of all the investigating detectives in the Boone County sheriff's department. When I heard that shriek from the hall on day one of my hospitalization, it was my mom, who almost fell flat into the arms of one of the detectives.

For the next three days, I revisited that night from a different perspective—that of the police officers. I thought about how they felt, envisioning a made-up exchange between two of them, replaying the scene over and over again in my mind.

"Let him die," shouts Officer Owens. "He doesn't deserve to be saved."

"Are you fucking kidding me, Owens?" yells Officer Gimble.

"You saw what he did. Let's let him bleed out."

Gimble pushes Owens out of the way and kneels down in front of my soon-to-be corpse. "If he's still alive, there's something we can do. I can't do nothing; it doesn't feel right. Give me the fucking tourniquet!"

While Owens was a product of my imagination, there actually was an "Officer Gimble," whose real name I learned after the case was closed. He didn't have to turn around and perform life-saving measures as I lay in the snow and bled all over his clothes. He didn't have to wrap my arm with a bandage. He didn't have to tourniquet my leg and put pressure on my stomach. That may sound cold, but some police departments don't require an officer to perform lifesaving procedures after inflicting a major injury, and even if I didn't mean to, I'd caused real harm of my own. How must they have felt going home that day and facing their families? How did they tell their spouses what happened? Where would they even begin? I made a detective cry, and six police officers were put on administrative leave for a mandated period of time because they'd had to discharge their weapons. I'm grateful to all of the officers who were at the scene, but if Officer Gimble ever reads this, I'd especially like him to know how profoundly I appreciate what he did for me.

• • • • • • •

Several months after my meeting with Harry and Boxer, I was finally ready to leave the hospital. I'd be under house arrest, only permitted to leave for medical, counseling, and attorney appointments, until my ultimate fate was determined. The bond for my release had been set at an amount significantly higher than the loan I would've had to pay back if I had simply quit ROTC. But at least I wasn't going straight to prison. Soon I'd be headed home with my mom and stepdad, and my trauma and fears for the future would, I hoped, exist only as a reflection in the rear-view mirror. For a split second I thought, *My life isn't in shambles.* I was just overjoyed enough to crack the first smile I'd made in about six months—and then my colostomy bag leaked all over the side of my stomach and onto the wheelchair.

Well, nothing new there. It had done this dozens of times before at the most inopportune moments. If and when my colostomy surgery was revised, I'd have another reason to smile. Until then, I needed to focus on my next challenge: reentering the world with a damaged body and a troubled mind.

16 HEALING IN SLO-MO

I WHEELED MYSELF to the garage door of our country home. It opened slowly, revealing a space that was much emptier than the last time I visited. A lot of equipment, large tools, and other items were missing. Had my mom and stepdad sold them off to help pay for the expensive decision I'd made?

When I entered the house, two puppies with a pedigree of pure energy greeted me. They were certainly excited to see me. Unfortunately, I wasn't able to fully interact with the only beings who wouldn't ask me awkward questions about how I'd ended up in this situation. They were contained within an enclosure to ensure they didn't pounce all over my injured body.

We maneuvered to the bedroom that was reserved for my stay until the courts decided what should be done with me. Within the room's generic white walls was a twin bed, a small TV, and clothes that had been packed neatly onto multiple shelves along with medical supplies. As I took in my surroundings, it dawned on me that I no longer had nurses and doctors to care for my daily needs. All of that was now on my parents. To add to my sense of unease, the bed was significantly higher than the ones I'd used in the hospital, and it lacked the levers that allowed me to reposition it so I could get in and out.

I called for my mother, and she assisted me onto the bed. I'd finally made it home, but I was still every bit as reliant on others for my survival as I'd been in the hospital. My mother would be responsible for most of my care while my stepfather worked extra hours day and night to help pay off the bills.

Getting to the dinner table was a slow, repetitive process similar to navigating to the rec room from my hospital bed. Moving from room to room and transferring to and from my wheelchair hadn't gotten any easier. But on the bright side, instead of being questioned at the end of my journey about the stupid things I'd done on the worst day of my life, my efforts were rewarded by a good meal with my family. Any home-cooked food would've been a nice change of pace from the hospital's typical frozen-and-reheated selections, but my mom had made shepherd's pie, one of my favorites. The flavor was more intense than I remembered, not because my mom had done anything new with the recipe but because it was different than what I'd become accustomed to over the last few months. It felt comforting that she'd thought to do this for me. I savored every single bite.

That night I woke up in pain. The meal that soothed my soul had also irritated my intestines, and the resulting diarrhea leaked out around my ostomy bag as I slept. I couldn't change the ostomy bag or clean it up by myself, and I had to scream for help.

Afterward, I had trouble going back to sleep. I lay there in the dark, humiliated, with grim thoughts about my future lurking in the crevasses of my mind.

• • • • • • •

Getting out of bed the next morning proved difficult. I attempted to heave myself up and failed. I tried to stay motivated, putting all my physical strength behind my efforts, but frustration got the better of me. My eyes shifted to a plastic water bottle on the bedside table, and I reached over to pick it up. It slipped through my weak fingers, fell to the floor, and rolled under the bed, soaking both me and the bed on the way down. I ended up asking my mother for assistance. It was going to be a long day.

First on the list of things to do, apart from the seemingly endless activities of daily living, was a primary care medical appointment. Since we lived in the middle of nowhere, this involved another long trip. More panting and struggling ensued as I attempted to move myself from the car into a wheelchair and through the office doors. The process was similar to the one right before meeting the detectives: left foot first, shift weight to the right, then lean over with the right arm and grab. "I can do it," I told my mother for the first time. "Stop." I managed to pick myself up after ten minutes. Now I only had to do these steps a hundred more times before they became easy.

The physician I'd come to see would, along with my mom, be responsible for coordinating all my physical and mental care from this point forward. I would need many more surgeries, physical and occupational therapy, and a lot of mental rehabilitation.

After looking at my file closely, Dr. Berger was speechless for a few awkward moments that seemed like hours.

"Were you depressed when you decided to move forward with this?" he asked.

Wow, we were jumping straight into this. I'd expected to start off slow, with the typical "how do you feel" questions. But then, those questions would've been a waste of time anyway. How could I have answered? "Well, I might be incarcerated, my arm may never fully heal, and I could defecate out of the side of my abdomen at any moment, showering your beautiful cheap carpet with undigested crap. Other than that, I'm great."I responded with a simple "Yes." I'd attempted to kill myself, so I must've been depressed, right? I didn't have the vocabulary to describe the situation any other way.

Dr. Berger threw more generic "how are you feeling" questions in my direction after my first response. "What is your plan to improve?" he asked. "Are you feeling the same way at all?" I gave answers that aligned with what a person on the road to recovery would say: *I should do such and so the next time I find myself in a similar situation. I'm doing fine, and I'm getting better.*

• • • • • • •

I was not fine. I was unhappy, and I was angry at myself. With the benefit of hindsight, I understood that when I'd felt sad, overworked, and stressed due to my circumstances at school, I'd brought those circumstances on myself. I could have stopped the events of February 18, 2015, at any time by simply saying no, and I chose not to. Although I couldn't quite articulate it yet, I had a sense that I hadn't even been clinically depressed at the time of my decision to kill myself—I did it because I was sad about my perceived inability to do anything constructive to solve my self-imposed problems. Now there weren't many good choices left to me, or to the family members who'd had no say in my original bad decisions.

I was still taking the antidepressants I'd been prescribed in the hospital. It's possible that they helped with my mood, but they also came with side effects, one of which was an uncontrollable urge to eat. I gained too much weight too quickly, which put a terrible strain on all of my abdominal wounds and made me depressed about yet another hit to my body image.

I didn't share much of what was going on in my head. In fact, I didn't communicate much at all—the most obvious outward sign that I needed help. In the past, I'd been outgoing and chatty. Now I was afraid of talking to other people. And I simply didn't feel like it after what had happened.

It was probably obvious to everyone around me that I needed professional help. The idea of seeking it out didn't appeal to me much, though. The last thing I wanted to do was talk about my feelings, and all that post-divorce family therapy back in the day had been a complete waste of my time. But I didn't have a choice: one of the requirements of my house arrest was that I see a therapist. My court-mandated counseling began about a month after my return home.

When I met with Jeff for the first time, I felt extremely spacey and disconnected, and I didn't really care for being there. He began with basic get-to-know-you questions: *Tell me your name.*

Where are you from? How are you feeling? What's your goal for these counseling sessions?

I wasn't particularly impressed with him. With a physique that wasn't up to my former gym-rat standards, something about the way he carried himself made me think he was just as lonely as I was. I couldn't tell you what led me to that conclusion, probably because it was bullshit. I still had a habit of projecting my own reality onto others. I looked everywhere for signs that other people suffered the way I did, that my own pain didn't make me weird or inferior.

Oblivious or indifferent to my misplaced judgment, Jeff turned out to be outstanding at his job. After his introductory queries he didn't bombard me with questions. He literally stared at me for two minutes, then said, "Talk about the first thing that pops into your mind—nothing more, nothing less."

I mumbled something about feeling lost and confused. I didn't understand how reality had brought me to where I was now.

He asked another question based on my response, probing deeper once he sensed I felt comfortable enough for him to do so. His unscripted approach felt personal and engaging, allowing me to open up on the very first visit. In the space he provided, I could safely relive my nightmarish experiences. I could even feel okay about sharing our deepest, darkest conversations with my mother when I was sent home with her.

During the first ten sessions, one of the things we spoke about in great detail was how the scars from my bullet wounds would attract attention that I didn't know how to handle. Jeff gave me techniques to employ if people made remarks about my disabilities or disfigurements (which they never actually did, but I was nervous about the possibility), or if I caught them staring at me (which they occasionally did). None of these techniques involved any kind of verbal response. He taught me to relax my core and breathe in and out when something made me anxious. He also sent me home with exercises that helped me practice interacting with others and not stress out if an uncomfortable topic arose.

• • • • • • •

"You keep staring at the right side of your stomach," Jeff observed around session twenty-three. Tell me why you're doing this."

"I'm just pulling down my shirt."

"No, you're not. You're looking at the bag. Why? You've looked at it ten times now."

Busted. "It's bothering me, and I can't stop thinking about it."

"Why are you so fixated on getting the colostomy reversed? You've been talking about it a lot," he said.

"Nobody wants this! Why would I want to deal with it?"

"When your mother took you outside last night after getting home and asked you what you would do if you couldn't get your colostomy surgery reversed, how did you react?"

"I told her I'd would try to kill myself again. I don't want to live with this. I couldn't handle it. I'd want to die again," I admitted.

A brief silence ensued.

"We've done all this work to get you to where you are now, and snap, just like that, you're willing to end it all so easily again?" Jeff said. "Are you just going to kill yourself if you lose a foot in a car accident, if you lose your hearing? You can't be perfect. No one is."

"Yeah, but I can't control getting into an accident."

"And you can't control getting old, either. If a situation gets hard, find a solution, don't run away from it."

When I got home, I wheeled into the guest room, lay down, waited for dinner, ate, and spent the rest of the night thinking about what he said until I fell asleep. Damn, he was right.

• • • • • • •

Weeks turned into months, and the months were full of activity. As I made progress on my mental health, eventually tapering off the antidepressants, I underwent multiple surgeries on my abdomen, legs, and left arm. I also got the colostomy reversed. The subsequent physical and occupational therapy was grueling; my mom took charge of that part of my recovery and put me through my paces like a drill sergeant.

Meanwhile, my attorneys worked tirelessly on my behalf. There were court hearings and a multitude of phone calls between myself, the legal team, and my parents. Friends, family members, and a number of medical professionals from various fields wrote letters to the court in support of me. I ultimately received one year of probation for every felony charge of wanton endangerment. If I violated my probation even once, my probation would be terminated, and I'd serve all of those years in prison. I resolved to make sure that I'd commit not even one violation of the agreement made with the State of Kentucky. No way would I jeopardize my second chance at life.

Finally, it was time for therapy session thirty-four, the final one, and I felt like it would be the most crucial. After all of the positive steps I'd taken, I realized, I was no longer depressed. Did that mean my trauma wouldn't affect me for the rest of my life?

"You've made a lot of progress," Jeff said. "Probably more than just about anyone would, given your situation. For the last few months, you haven't talked about the trauma of the event that transpired even once."

Wow, he was right. I'd spoken about that well into my fifteenth session, but my focus on it dwindled naturally until I stopped talking about it. I hadn't even ruminated on the events that day.

"But, just to confirm, I want to make sure . . . Are you avoiding discussing this, or do you truly feel less impacted by this than someone in your shoes typically would? You're smiling. I've not seen you smile once since you've come in."

I laughed as my mind inexplicably jumped to when I was a kindergartener, trying to curry favor with the cool kids. Why did I eat that worm?

17 REENTRY

WITH MY LAST therapy session behind me, it was time to start thinking about rejoining the world. The first step would be finishing my college degree. Before the events of February 18, 2015, I was only two months from graduating. Now that I'd gained the freedom to venture beyond my parents' front yard for activities other than seeing doctors, therapists, and lawyers, I decided to go back to IU. I'd received credit for all but a couple of courses I'd taken during what was supposed to be my final semester. Just two summer school classes stood between me and a diploma.

I was primarily using a cane to get around now, only switching over to the wheelchair occasionally when I got tired, and I'd recovered to the point where I could drive. On the morning of my first class, I took a minute to find my car keys, then climbed into my 2002 Pontiac Bonneville, a dirty old sedan with well over two hundred thousand miles on her. *Okay! Here I go, off to confront society.*

I turned the key, and a wild *uuuurrrggg* screeched in my ear. The car wouldn't start. Great. I'd set aside time to prep Bonneville and see if she purred, so I wasn't worried about being late to my first class yet, but it was an inauspicious beginning.

My mom rushed outside. After establishing that the sound she'd heard was my car and not half the garage being blown up in the midst of a B-2 bombing raid, she offered a solution. "Just take the van, don't crash it," she said. "I love you, be safe, and don't care about what other people think when you get there."

I did care, though. Not only was I about to interact with the outside world for the first time in well over a year, but I would also be going back to a place with people who knew me and were aware of my history. During the thirty-minute drive into town and onto campus, I attempted to talk myself off the ledge. *All right, so if there are twenty-six students in my class, and it's been a long time since I left, none of my graduated classmates should be there. I don't have to worry about knowing any of them.* I did the math on several other variables as well. *There's no way anyone could recognize me. I'm fine. Stop overthinking.*

The parking garage right outside the building that held the classroom I would attend was rather empty. That gave me a little more confidence; no way would I run into anyone who knew me. Approaching the door to the main entrance, I extended my hand, grabbed the knob, and turned it. *Phew, no one's in the hallway.* I took a hundred steps and reached the door on the far left, eleven minutes early for class.

Sweating, I pushed the door about an inch open and heard voices from inside the room. I recognized none of them.

Okay, do or die. I stepped back, paused, and breathed in for a second. *What am I doing? What am I doing?* I thought. There were only four or so voices. No way did I know any of them. *To hell with it! I'm opening the door.*

The first person I made direct eye contact with was a cadet I recognized from Army ROTC. He knew exactly who I was.

Well, this blows fucking skunk farts.

There were only five of us in the room and twenty-four chairs. I grabbed a seat that was three rows behind him in an attempt to break eye contact. He looked back and stared at me again.

What, dude? What do you want, bug eyes! Stop staring at me!

Then my training from therapy kicked in. "Hey, man," I said. He returned the greeting with a quick "Hey," and we didn't speak at all for the rest of the eight weeks.

I told my mom what happened when I got home. She replied, "Get over it. It's going to happen for the rest of your life. Better get used to it now."

18 GUIDANCE TO SELF-RELIANCE

MY FATHER WAS a strong presence throughout my recovery. The day I moved back in with my mother and stepdad, he called from his apartment in Arizona and asked me how it felt to be back home. From that point forward, he called frequently to check in.

I had an incredible support system in the aftermath of my suicide attempt, but my biological father occupied a unique niche in that system. He was literally the only individual who never sugarcoated anything or avoided the tough conversations. My friends and other family members cared deeply about my well-being and wanted to know how I was doing, but they felt protective of me and never crossed a line that they believed would transport me back to the dark place I'd inhabited when I almost died. I never even bothered asking my mom and stepdad if they'd sold off the stuff in their garage to pay for my medical and legal bills because they wouldn't have admitted it if they did.

While everyone else was repeatedly asking me how I felt and if I needed anything, my dad's questions didn't begin and end with my mental and physical health. His attitude was more, *So it happened. What are you going to do about it now?* Scouring my mind to help me find a way forward, he asked me to-the-point questions and made matter-of-fact statements. "What's your plan now? What are your next steps? You can't stay at your mother's and hide the rest of your life."

The solution-oriented way he articulated everything would appear soulless to an outsider if they'd heard our calls. But it was his way of showing he cared, and it was the push I desperately needed after I'd recovered enough for other people's constant expressions of concern to become annoying.

Shortly after I finished my classes at Indiana University, Dad grew increasingly anxious about obtaining information about my well-being. He called me more often, each conversation lasting less than a couple of minutes. He didn't seem worried about me, necessarily, but he frequently asked how I was doing. Finally, in late August, twenty-one grueling months since my attempted suicide, he requested that I sit down and have a serious call with him.

"I think you should move out here to Arizona," he said after answering on the first ring.

"Ummm, when did you come up with this idea?"

"It would be good for you," he replied, ignoring my question. "It's a huge city, and you'll have the opportunity to get back out there, meet people, and get a job. I'll help you."

"I don't know if I'm ready for a job yet. I don't know what my plan is right now." I shrugged and shifted the phone closer.

"Your plan is to come out here," he said. "Let's get you back on your feet and make you successful. It's not going to be easy, but you need to do it. You're an adult."

Unbeknownst to me, my father had been talking about my future for some time now with my brother Lucas, who thought a change of environment would be healthy. During all of our recent calls, my dad had been gauging my mental state, trying to figure out whether I would be happier and more productive if I stayed with him. Of course, not having been included in any of these discussions, the proposal felt sudden—like, hit-with-a-ton-of-cement-blocks-that-had-fallen-out-of-the-sky sudden.

Excuses and what-ifs filled my mind. How would I reintegrate back into society? It would be mortifying to have to explain to someone what happened to me if they googled my name. Was I really ready?

"Okay, I can do that," I responded hesitantly.

"Great, I'll get everything ready for your move. See you in November."

Despite my discomfort, I felt a sense of clarity that I'd been working toward in therapy. It would have been embarrassing to ask him for help. But instead of feeling offended that he'd offered it, I was glad he made it sound like I didn't have a choice. Apparently the indignant, arrogant part of my personality that had stopped me from seeking support back at IU was dissipating. I was able to summon the courage to admit to myself that yes, I needed it. Ten minutes after the call, my embarrassment over the idea of accepting his offer was replaced by a more constructive line of thought: *I would love it if you could help me figure out where*

I'm going wrong and provide me a place to stay while I get back on my feet. I'm glad I have you.

• • • • • • •

My entitlement to free caregiving and pats on the back ended the moment my plane landed at the Phoenix International Airport. As my father approached me at the baggage claim, I recognized the familiar "it's time to get to work" expression on his face.

Déjà vu set in as we parked outside of my father and stepmother's home twenty minutes from the airport. What might be missing from their home because they sold them to pay off attorneys? What sacrifices did they make to finance my legal fees?

"You need to get a job," Dad said as soon as I settled in. "Don't get comfortable."

"Wow, we're really rushing into this, don't you think?"

"No, we're not, I'll help you with the resume, but you're interviewing." I'd been in my new home for maybe an hour, and we were already attempting what I believed to be mission impossible.

"Step one, get a job," my dad continued. "Step two, get a new driver's license. Step three, organize your bills. We can talk about rent once you have the job."

"Can you give me a bit? I just got here?"

"Yeah, of course. With my help, it will take you a few months to get organized instead of a year. Let's get to it."

My father sat down with me and gave me tips on writing an excellent resume. When I checked that off the agenda, he had me draft a budget, make an extensive list of all I would need to accomplish by my move-out date, and engage in a plethora of other life-altering activities. This took less than a week. All of it!

If you haven't caught on by now, my dad doesn't take breaks, and if something needs to be done, he's typically the first to push toward a solution. He doesn't always say it in so many words, but his actions scream, *No, we need to do it now. We need immediate results!* In my teens, I pushed back on this way of doing things. I didn't recognize the importance of directing my motivation and drive toward worthy, attainable goals. If only I had listened when I was eighteen, I would've allotted more time to my studies, making me better prepared emotionally to get myself back on track after going one day without sleep. I would've said no, it's not in my best interest to agree to a fun activity or a request for help with a chore. I'd be able to explain why I couldn't do certain things and specify what I was capable of doing. I wouldn't have prioritized looking muscular and fit to the point where I was willing to take unregulated workout supplements that quickly altered the chemistry of my brain.

But now I'd been given a second chance. It was time to take the training wheels off once again. If I fell, I knew I had the ability to get back up.

19

INTO THE DEEP END

ENTERING THE WORKPLACE involved two seemingly insurmountable challenges. The first was finding anyone who would hire a convicted felon. The second was relearning how to interact with other humans. I had become a hermit since my suicide attempt, and I didn't know how to talk to people anymore.

Insurmountable challenge number one actually ended up being pretty easy to surmount. In less than two weeks after my arrival in Arizona, I came across several job opportunities. I printed out copies of my resume, brought them with me to the interviews, and explained my situation to each of the prospective employers. They showed not even a hint of concern about it. In less than two weeks, I started at a local car dealership. Selling cars wasn't my first choice—it involved tons of human interaction, I'd never done sales, and I had no idea what I was getting into. This would be a beast. But I needed the money.

I squared off against challenge number two, human interaction, when my new manager dragged me to what he called "the

Pit" on my first day. "You're going to meet the team, Jack," Mulligan said. Before I could correct his pronunciation of my name, he patted me on the back and continued pulling me along.

"Wait, what's the Pit?"

"You'll see." We continued to our destination.

"Hey Marky Mark, this is Jack!" Mulligan yelled as we passed him in the hallway. "Introduce yourself, Jack. Marky, follow me."

"Hey, uh, my name is Ja—"

Mulligan cut me off and guided me to the door that led to the Pit. This was going to be chaotic. I could tell.

The scene on the other side of the door lived up to my expectations. Rave music blasted from the speakers overhead, and rows of telephones lined dozens of desks. The ringing was nonstop, with phones being picked up and dropped left and right. It seemed eerily similar to a stockbroker call center but with a lot more swearing.

"Yo, Dan, grab the phone! It's that nasty bitch from Peoria," said a hefty gentleman.

"Fucking ass, what does she want?"

"I don't know, something about an oil filter you promised her."

"I didn't promise her shit. Fuck it, send her over."

"Welcome to your new home," Mulligan said. "Hey Marky, show him the ropes."

It was the ultimate social trial by fire. I was immediately thrust into cold calls, jumping from a setting where everyone was concerned about my well-being to a kill-or-be-killed battleground where I had to compete with sales veterans and outwit them. Despite all my progress, I hadn't believed I was ready to communicate with anyone outside my circle of immediate family members, medical professionals, and lawyers. Dealing with customers felt overwhelming, and my coworkers called me a pussy every time I stuttered on the phone. Not exactly the ideal environment for readapting to the real world.

Except, it kind of was. Forced to man up, I transitioned from total anti-socialite to hardened communicator real quick. While I wasn't great at sales, and I wouldn't feel completely normal when I talked to anyone for another two or three months, it took less than a week to retrain my brain to deal with stress, yelling, clashes with customers, and arguments with other salespeople—less than a week before my old personality rose to the surface.

Maybe a day or two after I'd hit my stride in terms of talking to people, my father was ready to move on to the next steps. "Great, you found a job," he said. "I'm giving you six months to move out. Oh, and you're also paying me $400 a month for rent."

Anger and confusion consumed me as they had before. I thought he was trying to make me upset. I wanted to harm myself. But these emotions dissipated quickly.

"Dad, I'm struggling. I need your help."

"It's not meant to be easy," he said. "You don't get a break just because you endure a traumatic life event. I care for you, and I want to see you succeed. I'll give you more tools to help. Just so you know, in less than three weeks, you accomplished more than you had in the last year and a half, and I'm proud of you."

"Thank you?"

"Your mother did a great job in Indiana—she helped you break out of your state of sadness—but now I need to help you financially. We'll get you there, bit by bit. Don't think about the time frame. Think about what we're going to accomplish in these six months."

He'd rehearsed this speech several times, I'm sure of it. My eyes shifted to my stepmother. "Do you agree with him?"

"Your father's right. You're making progress. Don't stop. We're both proud of you."

It felt as though I was being force-fed independence. But maybe it was just time I learned how to be an adult. My dad had wanted to help prepare me for the real world when I went to college, calling me all the time with advice about things like resume building, budgeting, and credit scores. *Here's a good way of doing this. Here's a better way to do that.* He'd handed me the keys to success, and I tossed them away because I was more interested in partying, hooking up with random women, and bodybuilding. Now he was giving me a second set of keys. Paying $400 for rent, $300 for food, and so on would teach me the cost of living, of surviving.

• • • • • • •

I began to improve at my job in a matter of weeks. Despite the clichés about dishonest car salespeople (which are largely accurate), I learned that you don't have to lie to customers to close a deal. Telling the truth and knowing your shit will get you a hell of a lot further. Still, I hadn't gotten good enough yet to earn the grand income that had been advertised to me. As grateful as I was for the opportunity to work at the dealership, living on my own with a commission-only job wouldn't be easy. How would I pay rent, feed myself, and make sure I could afford car payments?

As I worked to reach a place where I'd be responsible for my own financial, emotional, and physical well-being, I realized how lucky I was to have my parents in my corner. My mother had offered emotional support when I needed it most, placing value on comfort above all else as I stayed with her and Mark. Her job was to make me feel secure enough to be able to receive help from my father, whose job was to teach me to be a man and survive on my own. With their guidance, I learned that I needed to be thankful when others provided assistance while also understanding that I couldn't always rely on others for help. I needed to know how to identify problems early on, determine the catalysts, and immediately draft solutions. All of this would require a degree of humility, honesty, and awareness that I'd lacked before.

I knew now that I could do it. Having proven to myself that I could live in the world and hold down a job like anyone else, I'd begun to open my mind to new possibilities. I'd made a lot of mistakes, but I would never lose my new set of keys.

20 FLYING SOLO

IT ENDED UP taking more than six months to move out. Once I got settled at the dealership and my dad could tell that I wasn't just coasting, he was okay with giving me more time to save money before I got my own place. A year and three months after I started my job, I came across a new job opening. Another local dealership needed an internet manager—someone to handle all of the online leads that came in and to close deals with potential customers. The position was a step up, the company had a better commission plan, and with only six sales reps working there (as opposed to forty at my current place of employment), there would be less competition and more sales opportunities.

I applied. I got the job.

Now I was finally ready to rent a place of my own. But was anyone ready to rent to me? It didn't take long after I began my search to find out that most property management companies flag anyone who has a criminal record or a credit score of less than 620. Buying a home instead of renting would've enabled me to get around the background checks, but that wasn't an option. It would've taken another three years of putting money aside before I could afford a down payment.

But all was not lost. I discovered that the smaller an apartment complex is, the easier it is to get accepted—mom-and-pop owners tend not to utilize the property management companies that automatically deny certain applicants based on predetermined criteria. I spent the better half of a day roaming Scottsdale (population 250,000) and visiting complexes with fewer than twenty units each until I found one that would accept me. At a property fairly close to my new job, I spoke with the owner, described my situation, and was accepted right away.

• • • • • • •

Having put a deposit down on my own apartment, I needed to acquire stuff for it All I had to my name was a leased car, a few bags of clothes, an iron, and an ironing board. For this endeavor, I received some unexpected help from family. My aunt Genevieve and uncle Michel had moved to Arizona shortly after my father arrived here and convinced them it would be a much more pleasant environment than chilly Montreal. They called me after my father informed them of my move and offered to contribute various pieces of hand-me-down furniture, which I gratefully accepted. While the seams of the table legs and chairs brought to mind 1880s Victorian London—ugly and not exactly my style—I had zero complaints. Free was good.

To supplement my aunt and uncle's contributions, I took a quick trip to IKEA with my father and stepmother. They'd told me I would be paying for the furniture, but when we got to the checkout line, my father said, "I got this. You've worked hard. I'm happy to see where you are and how far you've gone."

A week later I took my first steps into the new place. While it wasn't as nice as my dad's, it was quaint, comfortable, and spacious, with enough room for everything I owned (which admittedly still wasn't much besides furniture). Located on a busy street in Scottsdale, it was also far from soundproof. The commotion outside seemed similar to what you'd find in New York. Cars swooshed down the road, constantly littering the dining room with noise. I closed the windows, sat on my couch, and took a deep breath. It was nice to be alone, to finally have breathing room.

My new job would start the following day. I got ready for it, doing the paperwork and putting my clothes away, leaving one outfit out for the morning. Nervous excitement filled my mind. This was my new life. I was fully independent now, and free of the shadows of my past. No more follow-up appointments with doctors regarding my physical health. No more waiting for a legal system to decide my fate or for a lab to do bloodwork checking for lead from bullet fragments. My mind was 100 percent clear, and I had the means to pay my own way, respond in a healthy way to whatever obstacles arose, and determine my own future. It could only get better from here.

EPILOGUE

MY INSTRUCTOR PULLED me toward the exit door on the left side of the plane, which had been open since takeoff. As I'd rehearsed during our tandem jump, I looked down and located the drop zone—the place where I was supposed to land. I remained there for a good thirty seconds, hanging out over thirteen thousand feet of air, waiting for my instructor's hand signals. When they came, I grabbed onto a bar inside the door, kicked my legs out, and faced in the direction the plane was flying.

Then I let go.

• • • • • • •

Ever since I gained enough experience to take a hill with confidence, I've felt the urge to test my limits. When I went skiing with my dad as a kid, he would always complain about how I wanted to go really fast even though my form wasn't all that good. If I wiped out, it would be while I was going ninety miles an hour in a straight line. But my interest in making the leap to extreme sports was initially inspired by the 1991 film *Point Break*, which I watched in my apartment at twenty-five years old. Johnny Utah's pedigree of surfing, snowboarding, and skydiving was badass. Bodhi, the thrill-seeking, boundary-pushing antagonist with zero fear of injury or death, seemed to be telling me to go for it, regardless of the consequences. The FBI agents—to me the movie's true antagonists—represented an attempt to quell my desire for excitement by imposing rules on what people could and could not attempt.

Sometime later, a random idea about learning how to skydive popped into my head. With these fictional characters (and real-life stuntmen) as my role models, I jumped right into it. My first solo descent, after the initial terror passed, was actually quite relaxing. Landing was the hard part. I had to flare brakes on the canopy and time it well to avoid dunking, dropping, and sliding aggressively on my ass when I hit the ground. The whole thing went off without a hitch. Since then, I've routinely engaged in activities like skydiving, extreme skiing (which encompasses backcountry powder, heli, and cat), mountain biking, rock climbing, and bouldering. Not bad for somebody who almost lost the ability to get out of bed.

That's not to say that all of my exploits have gone according to plan. One time, I skinned my left index finger across the ground after unintentionally performing the most incredible scorpion (a maneuver where you flip your body upside down while landing). It only bled a little, but the minor injury led to an infection, and I eventually had to get the very tip of that finger chopped off (technically, I now have 9.8 fingers). More recently, I got hurt in a skiing accident because I thought I was capable of performing a backflip off an icy fifty-foot ramp in Snowbowl, Arizona. Mid-jump, I looked down and to the left, realized I was still higher than the chairlift, and thought, *I'm not supposed to be this high up, still.* The friend recording me was kind enough to immediately drop his phone after I landed on my back and blacked out.

Jacques, you might be thinking, *you've already suffered so many serious injuries as a result of taking stupid risks. Why do you partake in these sports?* Fair question, as these tales of preventable mishaps make it sound as though I've simply replaced one set of risky activities with another. It's true that part of the appeal is getting out of my comfort zone. Every time I hike a mountain or hop on a plane or chairlift, I get the jitters. Overcoming them and making it to the peak or the ground feels amazing. And let's be honest, my ego is enormous. I tell myself that I look amazing doing it, even though I know most people don't care.

That said, I fully acknowledge my fear of dying now. I'm cautious. The key to staying safe is keeping it simple, not trying maneuvers that are beyond my current abilities, and being open to learning. My huge ego doesn't stop me from asking for guidance from people who know significantly more about what I'm trying to achieve than me. When I do fuck up and take too much of a risk, I reflect on what happened and learn from my mistakes. For instance, I bit off more than I could chew with that backflip in Snowbowl because I felt I was experienced enough to pull it off. But experience doesn't translate to rehearsal. If I'd scouted the ramp before jumping it, I would've realized that the ice at the top made it too dangerous.

In any case, believe it or not, my love for these sports isn't really about the adrenaline rush—it's about communing with nature. As an avid amateur skydiver, powder and downhill skier, and paraglider, I have an opportunity to interact with the natural environment in a unique way. Every time I stand at the edge of a cliff I've hiked to, or the top of a mesa I'm about to ski down, or the door of a plane I'm preparing to jump out of, I'm inspired by the terrain. The sky. The breathtaking mountains of the west and southwest. The pure, raw, humbling force of nature. I have a better appreciation for life now, and this is my way of showing it.

It sounds counterintuitive, but extreme sports bring more calmness to my life than excitement. When I do a backflip out the back of an Otter airplane, it feels as if I'm looking up at my past, leaving it behind. Honestly, when it comes to getting out of my comfort zone, jumping out of planes and skiing down mountains has been way less scary than writing my experiences down on paper and telling the entire world about my stupid mistakes.

• • • • • • •

Up until I was about twenty-six, I had no interest in telling people the truth when they asked about the scar on my left arm. "Oh, this?" I'd say before quickly changing the subject. "I was in a major car accident." Or, "I fell off a motorcycle." (I don't even own a motorcycle.) The most outrageous response I gave while trying to impress someone: "Yeah, I was bit by a shark." I persuaded myself that other people would find that convincing, as the jagged edges of the scar from my wrist down to my elbow resemble teeth marks.

A few factors eventually led me to entertain the idea of just being honest. One was associating with others who share my interests. More people than you realize get involved with extreme sports because of some prior life-changing event. I've met several individuals with even crazier stories than mine. They didn't hesitate to tell me their stories. Why couldn't I do the same?

Of course, it's sometimes not the greatest idea to launch into my whole story when the question comes up—for instance, if I'm talking to customers. In situations like that, I simply say, "It was a bad decision, a really stupid one." The funniest response I ever received to that answer occurred in the dealership showroom when I was closing a deal for a middle-aged couple on a preowned Honda Civic. The woman replied, "Yeah, guys are pretty stupid sometimes. Just look at my husband." I chuckled as she gave him a disdainful look. He had a pencil-length scarred abrasion on his neck that wrapped around the back of his spinal column.

"I got myself shot by the police," he said.

"Why?" I said.

As soon as the word was out of my mouth, I realized I'd been unprofessional. *Oh crap,* I thought. *Now he's going to get emotional, and I'm going to get fired for asking inappropriate questions.* Fortunately, neither of them were upset or offended. I spoke with the guy for another thirty minutes, until my boss reminded me that they were ready to sign paperwork in a finance office. Resuming my role as an internet manager, I walked the couple back towards the office. Halfway through the hallway, the man said, "I know you were shot too. I can tell."

He'd been shot several times when, in a drunken state, he threatened to kill himself with a knife, refused to put the knife down, and ran with it toward the police. One bullet severed a portion of his spinal column at the neck, leaving him unable to walk for three years. He met his wife two years later. They'd been together for twenty-four years when I met them. "On our third date," he recalled, "she asked me how I got the scar. I told her right there and then." He wouldn't have had his three children, now college graduates, if he hadn't been honest with her from the get-go. His story helped me feel more comfortable about telling mine.

Sadly, before that happened, I lost two friends who knew nothing about my past. I'd been too scared to share it with them. I kept thinking I'd put it off another week because I other things going on. Now I can't help but wonder—if I'd told them, would they still be alive today? Would explaining how I spiraled, and how my decisions severely impacted people who loved me, have been enough to deter them from taking their own lives? I'll never know because I was complacent and waited too long. In sharing all of this with you, my hope is that you can learn from my mistakes and choose better options than I did.

During the long struggle to regain my mental and physical health, I learned that I could push past fear to achieve my goals. While life doesn't always give you training wheels, sometimes falling off the bike teaches you how to get back up. If you land in a thornbush, you still have the ability to crawl back to the top of that hill. But at the same time, you need to know the difference between an acceptable risk and a foolish, pointless one. Sometimes courage means attempting something scary. Sometimes it means saying, "No. I can't. I'm not ready just yet." And sometimes it means asking for help.

I can't emphasize that last point enough. I've only achieved what I have today because of a tight-knit support system. The backbone of my success has been a willingness to accept the knowledge offered by others, from my parents to my therapist to my skydive and paraglide instructors. If you're in a bad place right now, look to people you trust for guidance, ask them explicitly for support, and listen to what they have to say. Don't be the person who tries to manage all the problems on their own until the problems become unmanageable. Because when I revisit my ordeal in conversations with strangers today, I can think of only three words to describe it: "That was stupid."

And if you've already done the stupid thing? Don't give up. As long as you're alive, you have the opportunity to make better choices. When I look back on everything I went through, I tell myself, "Yeah, that was stupid, but look at me now!"

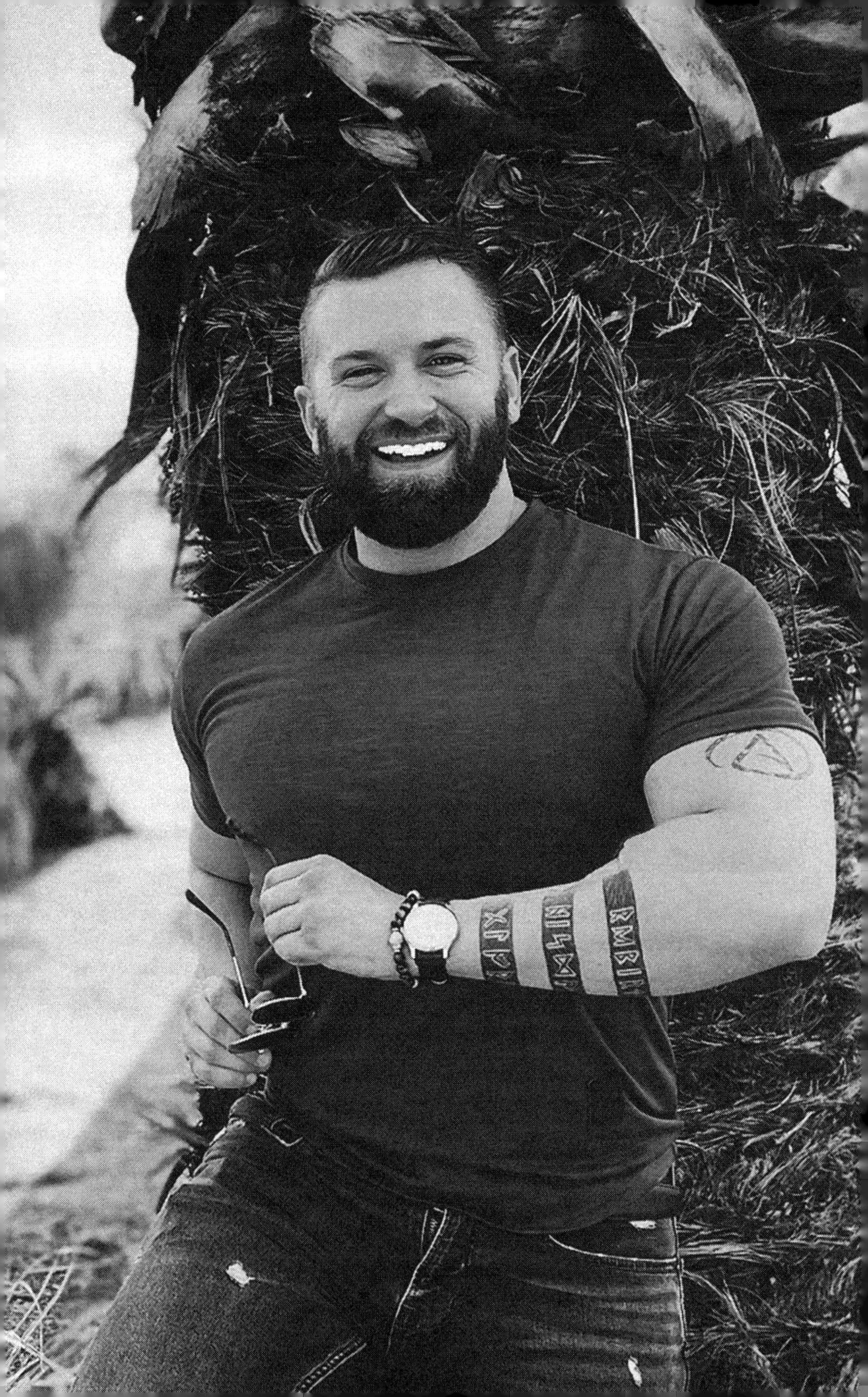

ABOUT THE AUTHOR

Jacques Poirier is an experienced extreme sports athlete, entrepreneur, Indiana University graduate, speaker, and advocate for the mental health community. His firsthand experience with mental-health issues drove him to write this captivating and inspiring memoir, which he hopes will encourage others to come forward and share their own stories.

The battle for mental health rages every day. You can join the fight against suicide and depression at

WWW.XTREMENOMAD.COM

Made in the USA
Columbia, SC
05 August 2024

12d16391-a800-426f-9d68-904c853da970R01